DR. CAS

The
Cannabis
Cure

Perfect wellness through the
powers of whole food,
raw cannabis extract.

Printed in the United States of America

ISBN: 9781931078351

Disclaimer: This book is not intended as a substitute for medical diagnosis or treatment. Anyone who has a serious disease should consult a physician before initiating any change in treatment or before beginning any new treatment.

To order this or additional Knowledge House books call: 1-800-295-3737 or order via the web at: www.knowledgehousepublishers.com

see also: www.cassingram.com

Other relevant Websites:
www.americanwildfoods.com
www.oreganol.com

To get an order form send a SASE to:
Knowledge House Publishers
105 East Townline Rd., Unit 116
Vernon Hills, IL 60061

Table of Contents

	Introduction	7
Chapter One	**The Chemistry of Hemp**	17
Chapter Two	**Ancient Uses, Modern Implications**	33
Chapter Three	**Recreational Use: a Panacea?**	39
Chapter Four	**Hormones, Sexual Organs, and More**	55
Chapter Five	**Marijuana, Good and Bad**	67
Chapter Six	**Cannabinoids to the Rescue**	87
Chapter Seven	**The CBD Revolution?**	97
Chapter Eight	**Medical Conditions**	105
Chapter Nine	**Neurological Conditions Resolved**	143
Chapter Ten	**Digestive Disorders and More**	175
Chapter Eleven	**A Cure for Addictions?**	193
Chapter Twelve	**Treating Hormonal Imbalances**	205
Chapter Thirteen	**Animals and Cannabis**	215
Chapter Fourteen	**The FDA and Hemp**	221
Chapter Fifteen	**Hemp and a Long Life**	231
Chapter Sixteen	**Conclusion**	249
	Appendix	257
	Bibliography	261
	Index	267

Introduction

There is a substance in nature which has exceedingly potent properties. It possesses properties which make it invaluable for a wide range of health conditions as well as the means for preventing such disorders. This is cannabis, also known popularly as marijuana. In this book what is described is medicinal marijuana, not the drug type that is smoked. It is the type which does not have hallucinogenic properties and will be hereby described as cannabis or hemp.

Regarding the non-hallucinogenic plant the term cannabis is synonymous with hemp. The now popular nutritional food, hemp seeds, is the seeds of the cannabis plant. Cannabis is merely the scientific name. It does not imply hallucinogenic properties.

In previous history hemp was used for a wide range of products, including the production of paper, clothes, and rope. Hemp rope is the toughest type known, and hemp-based paper, used, for instance, by Chinese and Islamic civilizations, is the sturdiest, longest-lasting ever produced. Books made from hemp paper are still extant today despite being 1000 years-plus old. In Europe such paper was also produced and used during the Middle Ages and, once again, is still extant through Medieval-era books. Yet, there are two kinds of cannabis, the food or industrial kind and also the addictive kind, the one grown for recreational use. Hemp, that is cannabis, is not evil to any degree and is, rather, of vast benefit upon humankind.

Even so, there is a form which is noxious. This is marijuana, the type raised as a hallucinogen. The regular smoking of such hallucinogenic plant matter is an issue of concern, as it does lead to negative effects, both upon the individual and society at-large. Like any other drug the continuous use of marijuana can cause tissue damage, while also having a derogatory effect on the psyche. In contrast, the smoking of hemp is not an issue, that is industrial hemp, as it is not hallucinogenic and does not have negative effects upon the body. No one can get high on its leaves. Botanically, it is a different plant and is entirely safe for human consumption.

Extracts of the hemp plant as natural medicines have vast value. Here, no one is suggesting it be smoked. Rather, the premise of this book is in regard to the internal consumption of this astoundingly valuable natural medicine and/or its use topically. It is fully established that hemp is one of the most nutritionally dense of all foods, being exceedingly rich in vitamins and minerals as well as protein. What isn't as well established is that the plant has countless numbers of other highly potent substances, phytochemicals, which find vast use in the treatment of human disease.

These phytochemicals exert properties which are of value in a wide range of conditions, including potentially deadly diseases. Widespread in nature these phytochemicals or their similars are found in the barks of trees, in the needles of evergreens, within a wide range of foods, and, extensively, in aromatic plants such as spices and herbs. Collectively, these substances are known by a variety of distinctions such as aromatic compounds, phenolic compounds, aromatic esters, aromatic terpenes, terpenoid compounds, and, of course, that key distinction, cannabinoids.

By implication cannabinoids are substances found, as would be expected, in cannabis. Yet, this is a short-sighted view. The fact is hemp is merely one of a number of plants rich in these compounds. There is a notable reason they are so widespread. For optimal health living beings, whether animals or humans, need the cannabinoids. Such beings have specific, deliberate systems for making use of these substances. Consider the human body. Here is found a specialized physiological system known as the endocannabinoid system. The prefix "endo" means within. The endocannabinoid system is within the body for a specific reason, which is to accept cannabinoid receptor activators. These activators help modulate the function of a wide range of elements, including the detoxification, immune, neurological, and endocrine systems.

One such key hemp-based phytochemical is the aromatic compound caryophyllene, also known as Beta-caryophyllene. This is classified as a terpene molecule or terpenoid. It is a substance which may be regarded as virtually miraculous in its powers. In its terpene fraction concentrated extracts of hemp, known as CO_2 extracts, are up to 60% Beta-caryophyllene by weight. Other dense sources of this novel compound include black pepper, particularly the novel West African type, echinacea, hops, basil, rosemary, sage, and oregano.

Terpenes are defined as "unsaturated hydrocarbons." The compounds are made up of what is known as "repeating isoprene units." In fact, life is made up of such chemical compounds. They are also defined as any of a group of "unsaturated hydrocarbons of the chemical formula $C^{10}H^{16}$, found in essential oils and oleoresins of plants such as conifers." Virtually all evergreen trees are rich in terpenes.

That makes sense. Has not everyone heard of "turpentine," which is just one such terpene-rich complex from pine trees? In fact, turpentine is the obsolete term for describing these compounds.

American Heritage Dictionary states that the commonly known nutrient beta carotene is a terpene. That makes sense when considering the name, carotene. It is close to caryophyllene. Another chemical term which describes these novel substances is sesquiterpene, of which Beta-caryophyllene belongs. Sesquiterpenes are among the most powerful natural therapeutic substances known.

Obviously, then, terpenes are largely food-like substances. In other words, they are entirely edible. Merely the products of plant biosynthesis, where carbon is fixed as a result of the interaction of sunlight, terpenes are found in virtually all plant foods. They are most heavily concentrated in vegetation, that is barks, leaves, the stalks of plants, berries, fruit, and vegetables. The densest sources of the caryophyllenes are aromatic plants such as cannabis and flavorful spices, also those various trees with much aroma, including those of the pine and fir families.

No one bans for human use pine or fir bark or for that matter natural spices. How, then, can an extract of hemp, in this case of its stalks, be considered anything other than fully legal, impossible to ban? Regardless, no doubt, the industrial hemp species, the type ultra-low in hallucinogenic compounds, is an invaluable natural medicine. This is largely because of the terpenoid molecules, the most predominant of which are the caryophyllenes. The caryophyllene group of compounds exert their powers on the same class of receptor sites activated by marijuana: the cannabinoid receptors. As a drug marijuana acts on two groups of receptors, known as CB1 and CB2. These receptors are the key to understanding cannabis' powers. They act to coordinate signals to key organ systems in order to maintain a state in the body known as homeostasis. The latter essentially means normalization and/or balance in bodily functions. CB1 receptors are responsible for the mood-altering effects, known as psycho-active effects. In contrast, CB2 receptor sites are the conduit for therapeutic actions such as the body's response to inflammation, pain, immune activation, and in the fight against tissue damage as occurs in hardening of the arteries, cancer, arthritis, and osteoporosis. Activation of these receptors is health-giving. CB2 receptor activation is devoid of psychoactive reactions.

CB2 receptors are found in a wide range of tissues, including the intestinal canal, thyroid gland, adrenal glands, ovaries, testes, liver, spleen, heart, kidneys, blood vessels, lymphatic cells, and bones. Of course, they are also found in abundance in the brain and spinal cord although to a much lesser extent than CB1 receptors.

This is an impressive representation for these receptors. It demonstrates how truly powerful CB2 receptor activators are: that they could exert such a wide diversity of beneficial effects. In this regard it has been determined that caryophyllene molecules have a highly direct action on these tissue receptors. This substance selectively binds to the CB2 receptor sites, activating it or reviving it, that is if it is burdened by overload or toxicity. The same is true of the majority of the other 60 or so hemp-based cannabinoids.

Since the 1960s scientists have been fully aware of the existence of these receptor sites, knowing that their activation is a key in disease treatment and prevention. The body, scientists know, have them there for a reason, and the primary reason, they presume, is for regulation. They also know that industrial hemp is the richest source of cannabinoid receptor site activators known.

Yet, what has been the focus of modern science? It has been to synthesize CB2 activators, essentially, synthetic forms of cannabinoids. Many of these synthetics now exist with a number of them fully patented.

While hemp has a great diversity of cannabinoids, here, researchers have been short-sighted. They have focused on single substances, such as cannabinol and tetrahydrocannabinol, or THC, instead of the synergistic whole. That's right, all the various cannabinoids work in a complementary way together. Single molecules, whether isolated or synthetic, are not the answer. Nor is neglecting one of the most prolific ones, Beta-caryophyllene, an effective approach. THC is the active ingredient of hallucinogenic marijuana. This has led to the production of synthetic drugs and/or isolates based on this compound. Yet, despite its potential powers and much positive results there are significant drawbacks to such an approach, including relapses, treatment failures, and the potential for side effects.

The sophisticated nature of these various cannabinoids is fully established. Yet, they are no match for the ultimate cannabinoid receptor activator. This is Beta-caryophyllene, one of the most powerful therapeutic substances known. A focus on this molecule changes the entire platform for cannabis therapy. This is because rather than a drug Beta-caryophyllene is a foodstuff, essentially a food-based phytochemical. In fact, in terms of foods or herbs the most potent receptor activators are the plants which are richest in this substance. All such plants are phytochemical-rich and, therefore, therapeutic power-houses. The densest food/plant sources of Beta-caryophyllene are as follows:

- CO_2 hemp extract
- wild rosemary
- wild oregano
- black pepper, particularly West African types
- clove buds
- hops
- holy basil
- celery
- carrots
- regular parsley
- Italian parsley
- Italian parsley root
- wild sage
- lime
- cinnamon

All such foods, spices, and herbs have positive actions on the endocannabinoid system. In addition, the barks of various trees, notably pine and fir, are dense sources of this compound. Consider what is seen, here, the human experience, historically and medicinally, with such spices, herbs, and foods. These are among the most aromatic, intensely flavorful of all plant complexes known. It is the various caryophyllene molecules which are largely responsible for the intensity of these flavors as well as odors. Beta-caryophyllene and its sister molecules may well be the most medically important of all substances known, a discovery set forth in this book for the first time.

Relatively few foods and herbs are super-rich in this crucial terpene. That is why the above list is so important, because it demonstrates the densest sources known which can be readily consumed. Curiously, regarding people all over the world the listed foods, herbs, and spices are among the most popular of all. Who hasn't enjoyed the healthy feeling of eating carrot and celery sticks? Moreover, all people love oregano as a flavor-enhancer, and many people are major users of black pepper. A standard in the health-giving Mediterranean diet parsley is highly popular as a food flavoring and food on its own. The flavor of basil is enticing and highly warming. Consider lime; who doesn't enjoy the robust flavor it adds to virtually any food or beverage? Sage is less popular among Westerners, although it is unsurpassed when used in the cooking of liver and poultry. Wild sage tea is commonly consumed by long-lived, healthy mountain villagers of Greece and Turkey. Regarding cinnamon and cloves there is no need to reiterate their popularity, whether in ancient times, the Middle Age era, the Victorian age, or modern times.

So, it is clear. Whether deemed hemp or cannabis this plant is a food-like complex. In the wild deer browse on it. Birds relish the seeds. Insects feast on the nectar. The components of cannabis are highly similar to those found in common foods and spices. The cannabis plant is a blessing to humankind. Let us learn its chemistry, nutritional density, medical uses, and far more in order to understand it and take maximum advantage of it. No doubt, it will prove to be a cure for all those who are desperate to improve their health and to reverse that oppressive trend of the onset of degenerative disease.

Chapter One

The Chemistry of Hemp

The name of the hemp plant, botanically, is Cannabis, that being the genus name. The species name is *sativa*. The other common species is *indica*, derived from its source, India. The terms hemp and cannabis will be used interchangeably. In contrast, the hallucinogenic type, that is the type that has hypnotic powers, will be referred to as marijuana.

It seems that some people can't get over the term cannabis. Somehow, they think it is bad: that it means pot. How can this be the case? It is merely its botanical identification. Pot or marijuana is bred to be hypnotic. Otherwise, no one would use it. Yet, the marijuana plant, too, is cannabis. Here, the type which is described is the industrial type, which is free of intoxicating powers to any degree. Cannabis is a descriptive term, because it identifies the original, non-intoxicating plant with vast medicinal powers, while also being used to describe the intoxicating variety, often leading to confusion.

Hemp is a terpenoid plant

Let us revisit the terms cannabinoid and terpenes, or terpenoid, because here is where the true powers, as well as sophistication, of the plant are found. Of the nearly 500 different compounds found in hemp some 60-plus are cannabinoids, and virtually all these molecules are terpenes. As published by R. Brenneisen in *Marijuana and the Cannabinoids* the term cannabinoid represents a group of chemicals which are phenolic compounds, more correctly, terpene-phenolic combinations known as terpenophenolic compounds. The description of these substances is important, because it explains the wide-ranging therapeutic powers of this plant. The substances are highly aromatic and account for the unique smell of cannabis but also those prominent aromas of other cannabinoid-rich plants such as spices, parsley, and celery. It is all the handiwork of the creator to make the food more appealing while also creating the necessary defensive mechanisms within the foodstuffs to protect them from pests and microbes.

Some 200 terpenes have been found in cannabis, which is a massive amount and makes the plant the most diverse source of these substances known. Only a few of these odoriferous, oily substances appear in sufficient quantities to be medicinally important. Here, it is crucial to realize that the density of terpenes varies considerably from strain to strain. Ideally, in the terpene fraction the medicinal complex should contain some 40% to 50% Beta-caryophyllene in extract form, while weaker forms may be as low as 5%. It is this terpene which is the major odor source for cannabis.

This variation in the density of this compound impacts not only the therapeutic value but also the odor and taste. The range of flavors of cannabis is extraordinary. No other plant known matches the cacophony of smells and tastes available. Caryophyllene is a sesquiterpene. This type of molecule is larger than the typical type of terpenes, known as monoterpenes. Examples of monoterpenes include pinene, limonene, and myrcene. While these are also medicinal, Beta-caryophyllene is different. Technically, it is a condensation of two benzene rings plus other structural components. It is known chemically as a bicyclic sesquiterpene. The prefix 'bi' indicates two, therefore, the two phenolic rings.

There is another reason it is unique among all cannabinoid chemicals. This is because it contains a specialized chemical component known as a cyclobutane ring, a rarity in nature. This ring component gives the compound unique chemical properties as well as a novel capacity for penetrating tissues, notably fat- or lipid-based tissues such as brain and nerve matter.

The compound is commonly found in the essential oils of numerous plants. Particularly predominant in spices and herbs, the richest known sources include cannabis along with black pepper, rosemary, hops, and wild oregano. For the human body here is the key regarding this novel molecule. The psychoactive element THC activates specifically the CB1 receptors, the ones that induce hallucinogenic responses. This is never the case with Beta-caryophyllene. It only activates the CB2 receptors, which are not associated with the marijuana high. In fact, in many respects CB2 activators antagonize the hallucinogenic effects of marijuana, as well as other drugs, like cocaine, and are, therefore, useful in their detoxification.

In contrast to isolated or drug-like forms Beta-caryophyllene is entirely safe for human consumption. In fact, a derivative of it, caryophyllene oxide, is used as a common food flavoring. Incidentally, since it is the main compound accounting for the strong, unique smell of marijuana caryophyllene oxide is used to train the smell of drug-sniffing dogs. The fact that in some cultivars Beta-caryophyllene and its related compounds accounts for in the terpene fraction some 50% of the volume is highly revealing, demonstrating the enormity of its value and power. Yet, incredibly, the research community largely neglected it. Instead, there has been a great deal of focus on cannabidiol. The substance has been extensively synthesized and is the basis of a number of drugs. However, in many respects Beta-caryophyllene is far more important, medically. Yet, ultimately, all 60-plus cannabinoids and various terpenes work together to account for hemp's medicinal powers. Clearly, Beta-caryophyllene is one of the most premier of these cannabinoids.

In the 21st century the molecule has become the subject of significant scientific studies, for instance, the work of a team of investigators with the United Arab Emirates University. It was these investigators who determined that rather than cannabidiol or THC it is the highly complex, sophisticated Beta-caryophyllene, which is *the premier hemp-source anti-anxiety and anti-depressive agent.* Publishing in the *Journal of Physiology & Behavior* they determined that the molecule has significant antidepressant actions and is also highly potent in reversing anxiety. These effects were directly a consequence of the action of Beta-caryophyllene on the brain's CB2 receptors. The results were held as highly significant. Even so, this may explain the common report by marijuana smokers of the anti-anxiety and stress-relieving actions of the drug. In fact, according to a 2013 report in *Trends in Pharmaceutical*

Sciences investigative studies have demonstrated that the primary reason for using cannabis is a result of "its ability to reduce feelings of stress, tension, and anxiety."

Yet, today, what is commonly done? Drugs and also plant extracts are made with the focus on cannabidiol alone. In fact, some marijuana-based drugs consist exclusively of this molecule, whether as a natural extract or synthetic copy. This is a highly erroneous approach. Who is to say which of the 60-odd molecules is most important? How can science fully determine the interactions of these widely diverse molecules and any synergistic or complimentary actions they possess? Moreover, what about the intelligence of raw nature, the balance, the unknown? All this is corrupted through the standard medical approach, the creation of isolates, refined extracts, and/or synthetic versions. This is why it is necessary to consume rather than an altered version the unprocessed whole, where all the various cannabinoids can be found in unison. This will provide the most potent therapeutic effect with the least opportunity for untoward reactions or side-effects.

It is always this way. Science deems a certain substance the active ingredient without any absolute basis. That becomes the trend, and all the other ingredients are secondary, if not being neglected altogether. Even in the herbal medicine business isolates are often the focus instead of the unprocessed, unaltered complex. That is certainly the case with the Beta-caryophyllenes, which rarely are discussed in the standard pro-medical cannabis circles.

Note researchers from ETH Zurich and Bonn University this substance has "largely been ignored." In fact, according one of the lead investigators of this group, J. Gertsch, no one knew about it until, incredibly, 2008. Yet, it has now been found in scientific studies to have "remarkable pharmacological effects."

One such pharmacological effect as determined by the Zurich and Bonn researchers is its antiinflammatory actions.

Gertsch makes a most crucial point. The molecule has a highly different structure than any of the other cannabinoids, being a novel phenol-based terpene. Investigators determined that this substance may well be the most crucial and powerful of all cannabinoids. This was by demonstrating, categorically, that Beta-caryophyllene directly attaches to CB2 receptor sites. In their study they induced inflammation in mice in a standard medical procedure where the paws are caused to become swollen and inflamed. Beta caryophyllene was administered, and the results were astounding. The swelling was reduced by some 70%. This action was proven to be directly due to the binding of the molecule on the endocannabinoid CB2 receptors. Yet, incredibly, it also works independently of such sites as a potent antiinflammatory agent and antioxidant.

It is reasonable to say that the investigators were fully astounded by the powers of this substance. Gertsch, for instance, found the actions of Beta-caryophyllene to be so impressive that he believes that it will eventually be turned into a drug-like substance, in this case to "heal certain forms of inflammation." The animal tests were so impressive that he also indicated that it will be instrumental in the treatment of chronic illness, including arthritis, hardening of the arteries, and even cirrhosis of the liver.

It all demonstrates the ultimate power of nature and also the innate powers of the human body. What a neglected area it is, that is this arena of internal signaling within the nervous system, the one controlled by both the internally produced cannabinoids and those arising from the diet. No wonder the health-giving properties of hemp, oregano, basil, hops, rosemary, and black pepper, the densest sources of Beta-caryophyllene, are so legion. Other top sources of this novel substance in percentage of the distilled essential oil are as follows:

*   West African pepper, that is pepper guineense (up to 58%)
*   clove buds (up to 19%)
*   cinnamon oil (up to 8%)
*   black caraway (up to 8%)

This substance is also concentrated in the distilled oils of wild oregano, rosemary, clove buds, and sage. Even so, of special note is West African pepper, also known as Ashanti Pepper and Pepper Guineense. Known also as uziza seed it is used traditionally as a natural medicine. It is no surprise that it is a folk remedy for arthritis and other inflammatory conditions. Says Dr. Paul Haider in his article *Ashanti Pepper, a Pepper with Healing Properties* the spice is "great for healing" damaged tissue and is especially used for "muscle pain, GI distress, and gas" and also for "improving memory,..." This correlates directly with the expected consequences of CB2 receptor activation. It has also been found that these peppers aid in the immune response and may also play a key role in restoring fertility. According to local investigators the pepper has the ability to raise sperm counts in infertile males. It is also an ideal medicine for intestinal complaints, and this is held to be a consequence of its germicidal powers. All this is largely the result of the rich Beta-caryophyllene content.

Consider the facts at-hand. Basil, wild oregano, wild rosemary, cinnamon, cloves, peppers, parsley, cannabis, and hops are all extremely dense sources of Beta-caryophyllene Yet, they are also historically and in the domain of modern science bona fide natural medicines. Let the world realize it, which is the fact that people can get well with such foods, spices, and herbs, largely as a result of the powers of that active ingredient, Beta-caryophyllene. After all, it was Gertsch who showed that it has a multitude of invaluable powers, including antiinflammatory, antioxidant, anti-cancerous, and local pain-controlling or anesthetic actions. Clearly, this natural, and ubiquitous compound is a superior type of natural medicine, far superior to synthetic cannabinoids. Regardless, all caryophyllenes are cannabinoids, no exceptions.

No wonder, then, the receptors for cannabinoids are among the most abundant in the human brain and are also expressed in nearly every other tissue and cell. Their abundance and diverse placement proves their immense value, strategically. Clearly, the creating Being made these receptors as signal activators and then produced the foods, herbs, and spices that are operative to facilitate them.

They truly are there for a reason. Gertsch and his group publishing in the *Proceedings of the National Academy of Sciences* demonstrated the immense powers of the Beta-caryophyllenes and was the first to deem them "dietary cannabinoids." Caryophyllene, he noted, is a "widespread plant volatile" and is a common constituent of the essential oils extracted from herbs and spices, while also being a major component of cannabis. In his research he revealed that the body has a high affinity for this class of compounds, which have their own docking sites on a number of cellular systems, particularly within the brain, liver, immune cells, kidneys, and bones. When the molecules bind to these docking/receptor sites, they cause the influx of calcium into the cells, among a wide range of other actions. It is rather incredible that such dramatic actions result from the interaction of these aromatic compounds with the cells in a fashion impossible to duplicate with any synthetic substance. White blood cells are directly activated and modulated through these interactions, while pro-inflammatory chemicals, known as cytokines, are reduced. White blood cells are, therefore, able to go about their job without inducing so much reactionary consequences. In other words, the inflammatory response of the immune system is modulated.

It has also been demonstrated that the caryophyllenes have significant anti-toxic powers. When test animals are exposed to noxious agents, such as carrageenan, which induces both inflammation and edema, oral caryophyllene halted the reaction.

Other key components in hemp

There are a number of other novel components in hemp, all of which possess medicinal properties. Myrcene is a sedative, pain-modulating agent, and muscle relaxant as well as an antiinflammatory compound. A major terpene in citrus, limonene, is a significant cannabis component. It functions as an immune potentiator and natural germicide. It is also a highly potent anti-tumor agent and has been shown to aid in the destruction of breast and colon cancer cells. Taken daily, it is preventive against a wide range of cancers. Furthermore, the terpene has also been found to aid in the dissolution of gallstones, while also reversing gastrointestinal reflux.

Certain cannabis strains contain a novel terpene known as linalool, also a prominent compound in lavender. Linalool is an anti-anxiety agent and is a strong anticonvulsant. It also acts as an antidepressant, aiding in serotonin metabolism. Topically, linalool has a strong action on skin diseases, aiding in the healing of acne, eczema, and burns, while preventing scarring.

CO_2 extract: a therapeutic powerhouse

The ideal way to gain the benefits of the hemp plant, that is the herbal part of the plant—the leaves, stalks, and flowers—is through a whole food extract. An extract implies that some element must be used to facilitate the extraction. Thus, in many instances alcohol and even more noxious solvents, such as butane, that is lighter fluid, and hexane, in other words, gasoline are used. Residues of these solvents have been known to intoxicate people. Ideally, extraction should be achieved without the use of such noxious substances. This is accomplished through a specialized extraction method known as supercritical CO_2 extraction.

CO_2 extraction is absolutely safe. In fact, because such extracts are fully health-reviving, this type of extraction is commonly used in the food and beverage industry. For instance, Drake Dorm in *CO_2 Extraction* notes that it is used in the production of soft drinks and in the removal of caffeine from coffee beans to make decaffeinated coffee. Therefore, it is the favored extraction method for the food industry. In contrast to alcohol, butane, and hexane carbon dioxide is a non-toxic, entirely natural solvent. When hemp stalks are treated with this, the result is a highly pure, unadulterated golden-colored paste loaded with phytochemicals and flavor.

The endocannabinoid system: a review

The endocannabinoid system is perhaps the most important functional system in the human body for creating ideal health. It does so by upholding good health and maintaining it, a process known as homeostasis. Too, it is the functional entity that is based on two elements: receptor sites and compounds which bind to and activate these sites. This system regulates key functions in both human and animal tissues. It is, essentially, a creator of signals that then go on to influence crucial internal organs, like the brain, spinal cord, heart, kidneys, immune system, hormone system, and more. Moreover, in all such organ systems it creates a highly sophisticated state, one that can be deemed, essentially, one of being on autopilot, which D. Sulak in his article *Introduction to the Endocannabinoid System* deems 'maintenance,' that is "the maintenance of the internal environment." This is so that it remains "stable" despite any fluctuations or disruptions from the internal or external environments. It achieves the creation of stability in the human cellular and organ systems. What could be more compelling than that?

The scientific world, being young at understanding this system, is surely astounded at the findings. Consider it, and do so carefully. Notes Sulak the endocannabinoid component is the balancing act of the human body. The cannabinoids, he states, perform this balancing act "at every level of biological life..." This implies that it holds sway over the prevention of virtually all diseases, as disease states are nothing other than gross imbalances.

It also holds the keys to prevention, even the achievement of a long, disease-free life. The most essential element of this according to scientific studies is continuous cleansing within human cells and organs. He gives the example of a process of self-cleansing known as "autophagy." This is the process where a cell holds within it some of its components to be purged and/or recycled. It's like cleaning out the filth or decaying matter in an old house. In purging it is a kind of self-digesting process. It allows cells to live as long as possible and also helps keep them from degenerating. It is all mediated by the endocannabinoid system. Furthermore, it means that the endocannabinoid system is the living being's most sophisticated recycling system known. For this reason alone people should be taking a whole food cannabinoid supplement.

Imagine the consequences if that system is defective or deficient. What will happen to those cells? They won't be able to cleanse themselves, to renew, or revive. There will be chaos in all the body. Toxins will accumulate to a degree of no return. As a result, the cells will degenerate and become cancerous. All this is prevented by a regular and adequate intake of cannabinoid complexes.

Yet, the system, notes Sulak, also targets cancer cells:

> It (that is the endocannabinoid system) has a deadly effect on malignant tumor cells, causing them to consume themselves in a programmed cellular suicide. The death of cancer cells...promotes homeostasis and survival at the level of the entire organism.

Nothing could be more astounding than this.

The ultimate proof of the powers and necessity of this system is actual biosynthesis within the human body. The body makes its own cannabinoids, synthesizing them from the fatty acid arachidonic acid. It then uses them as signaling molecules for the normalization of cellular function and also to deal with potentially damaging insults.

It is not, though, like a heart that pumps, lungs that breathe, or kidneys that excrete. No one realizes the system exists; it is that subtle. Moreover, who realizes that it is being influenced by what is eaten and consumed and what is not eaten and consumed? Yet, the existence of this system explains the resilience against disease of certain elements of the animal kingdom, as well as a number of primitive societies, whose diet is relatively rich in the compounds. Incredibly, until well into the 20th century the endocannabinoid complex was virtually unknown. Yet, the most mundane, basic functions are under it's control. If a person forgets, takes a nap, sleeps at night, sits down to relax, eats, and/or drinks, or merely attempts to find a modicum of balance in his/her life, such a one has done so through their endocannabinoid system.

Natively, the body knows this. That's why it produces its own cannabinoids. While it is known that a number of these exist only two have been identified to date. These internally produced cannabinoids are anandamide and 2-arachidonoylglycerol (2-AG).

CB2 receptors; how it all works

Specialized receptor sites on the cells, the CB2 receptors are found on countless cells of the body. Their purpose is to help regulate and balance cellular functions. These receptors are found in a high density in the immune organs, the organs of detoxification, the bones, and also in the brain and spinal cord. Activation of CB2 receptors has been shown in scientific studies to stall the progression of diseases of the nervous system. Yet, it is not just the nervous system which houses such receptors. These key complexes are found in multiple organ systems, including the cardiovascular, endocrine, immune, skeletal, skin, and liver-kidney systems.

In fact, these receptors are found to in a larger density in the immune system over all other organ systems. In the brain the main CB receptors are CB1. The receptor sites are based on specialized protein structures which are specific for receiving cannabinoids. The cannabinoids themselves are lipid molecules or, more correctly, phenolic and terpenoid compounds. Medically, these molecules are called lipid mediators.

CBD oil versus whole, raw extract: Which is better?

No doubt, the buzz in the cannabinoid world seems to be in regard to "CBD." Just what is this? Has anyone taken the time to truly analyze it? In fact, it stands for cannabidiol. This compound is merely one of some 66 cannabinoids found in whole food hemp extracts. When searching this abbreviation on the Internet, all manner of information is found. It is also determined that this is a most costly form of cannabis supplement, far more so than the whole, crude, unprocessed extract.

Despite the powers of cannabidiol or CBD such an isolated compound or concentrated extract is not the same as the whole. A truly whole food, raw cannabis extract contains CBD but also all the other cannabinoids plus dozens of other substances. CBD oils focus on the highly aggressive cannabidiol compound. This substance is so powerful that in an isolated form it can cause untoward effects. These effects include muscular heaviness, almost a sense that the limbs and body are too heavy to move. It can cause a person to feel too calm, almost apathetic. Those who consume it might "space out," not knowing what they did or when they did it. While none of these symptoms are dangerous, they are not desirable. Moreover, they do not occur through the intake of the whole, unprocessed crude extract.

CBD is different than the whole, crude, raw hemp extract. The latter contains rather complex molecules that operate in a sophisticated, steady-state fashion within the body. In contrast, CBD is a smaller molecule that has rapid actions. It should never be concentrated or isolated. It is too powerful for this. Thus, it should merely be consumed as part of the whole oil complex.

The fact is CBD oil can prove in some people to be too aggressive. In nature cannabidiol is never alone. In fact, no single cannabinoid should be taken as an isolated substance. Consider wild oregano oil. It has some 30 different key compounds, all of which work together synergistically. Does it make sense to isolate only one compound, like carvacrol, or to concentrate it at the expense of all others?

In addition to CBD and 60-plus other cannabinoids the whole leaf/stalk extract also contains sterols and waxes. These sterols and waxes are never found in isolated CBD oil. This is a true detriment, since these substances are essential for the health of all cells. It is the sterols and waxes that are needed to rebuild cell membranes, including, in particular, the membranes of the brain cells. This is why the hemp-wild oregano CO_2 extract is so ideal. All the components naturally found in the hemp and wild oregano plants are found in such a supplement. If God made it within the plant, it is there for a sound reason: no exceptions.

The raw juice: organic acids and more

Since hemp is an edible food, so is the raw juice. This juice is extracted from the young growing leaves. It is a most dense source of nutrients and is packed with minerals, vitamins, flavonoids, organic acids, essential oils, and rare trace elements. It is a particularly dense source of magnesium, which is highly needed by the human body. A deficiency of this mineral is one of the most common deficits known. Rich food sources of this mineral are relatively rare. Both the juice and hemp seeds are particularly exceptional sources.

The raw juice is one of the most ideal forms of cannabis, since it has no hallucinogenic compounds, that is there is nothing in it that could make a person high. It is also highly therapeutic, which is related directly to the raw, unprocessed nature of such a fresh production.

The fresh extract contains all the cannabinoids. In such a raw form these cannabinoids are highly biologically active. These are known as "acid" forms of these compounds. These acids, also known as organic acids, are highly sophisticated in their actions. They act as cleansing agents, inducing a strong detoxification response in virtually all tissues of the body, including the joints, skin, liver, kidneys, bloodstream, and more.

It is important to keep the juice in a raw state. It must never be cooked or heated in any way. Heating causes a reaction known as decarboxylation, which increases the THC content of the juice. The raw juice is highly vulnerable to this. Thus, it must be kept stabilized at all costs. This is achieved by the addition of Preservitol, which prevents such decarboxylation and also maintains the juice in a raw state.

Chapter Two

Ancient Uses, Modern Implications

What is the documented history of the marijuana plant? That history is highly significant, proving that it was used continuously as a food, drug, textile substance, and far more. About 10,000 B.C. the first recorded use of hemp was established based on ancient textiles found in Turkey. By 6000 B.C. the seed and seed oil were being used in China, while at 4000 B.C. hemp textiles were common throughout the Orient. By 2000 B.C. the first hard evidence for its use, medicinally, was in China, recorded by Emperor Shen Neng. At the same time in India, about 2000 B.C., ritual use was documented and it was mentioned in Hindu scriptures as "Sacred Grass."

In the 7th century B.C. a Persian religious text listed it as *bgang* or the "good narcotic." At about this time hemp seeds were found as offerings throughout tombs in the civilized world. The ancient Egyptians used cannabis to treat tumors, a significant discovery now proven by modern science. An ancient Egyptian text from the 2nd century called *Fayyum Medical Papyrus* contains the earliest known record for the use of this drug as a cancer medicine. About 100 B.C. hemp fibers were used in China to make paper. By the beginning of the A.D. era its use with spices and salt was determined through analysis of tomb remnants. About 50 A.D. the Roman-era author Pliny the Elder mentions the properties of cannabis as an effective analgesic, while Plutarch, about 100 A.D., describes its use as an intoxicant. Dioscorides mentioned it, listing it as an herbal drug. Later, in the 2nd century Galen prescribed it for the treatment of a wide range of conditions. In the 3rd through 4th centuries the herb gained favor for use in pain relief and sedation, being used to ease the pain of childbirth and also as a surgical anesthetic. In adopting from the Greeks during the Islamic Empire the drug was used by surgeons to fully sedate patients. This was in order to prevent them from experiencing post-operative pain, a special form of the drug was used to sedate them to be in a state as if asleep for up to a week. This is curious, considering the strict mandates in Islam against intoxication. It demonstrates the liberality for the discovery of marijuana when medically necessary, just like the use of opium derivatives not for mere recreational use but as potentially therapeutic drugs.

By the 10th century A.D. the use of hemp rope, as well as sails, in shipping was commonplace. However, with the passing graduation of years patterns of abuse developed. The toxicity of the drug was described, with Islamic authors warning of its potential dangers. It was in the 11th century A.D. and afterwards when hashish was apparently invented. Its use spread throughout the Middle East. In the *1001*

Arabian Nights hashish's intoxicating and aphrodisiac properties are described. Yet, this is not an endorsement of its use by the Islamic faith, quite to the contrary. It was the Prophet Muhammad in his wisdom who warned his followers of the danger of intoxicants, stating that they are all banned. Put simply, he said, *"Every* intoxicant is prohibited." This includes alcohol, heroin, codeine (taken for intoxicating purposes), amphetamines, LSD, cocaine, and, of course, marijuana.

The nature of his prohibition was explained by later scholars, who said banned substances are all those which corrupt human health, specifically by causing excessive relaxation and somnolence: that is corrupting the potential for productivity. Scholars deemed intoxicants any substance that causes the inability to function: muscularly and through the nervous system. Even so, as a drug marijuana was never consumed by the early Muslims. It simply did not exist at the time. Its widespread use came centuries later when an empire based on Central Asia, the Tartar Empire, was established. Even so, prior to this popular introduction Ibn Taymiyah said that in Islam there can be no doubt that it is banned, as the use of any psychoactive intoxicant is disallowed. This prohibition, of course, is in regard to the recreational use for purposes of getting high. There is no hard ban on its use as a medicine under a physician's prescription. Even so, let it be said, here, that the smoking of commercial marijuana is a most inferior drug, as it does create the potential for addiction. People may even use this as an excuse to gain the high. For medicinal purposes it is fully sufficient to use the legal, non-psychoactive type.

Yet as it became more widespread physicians of the Islamic Empire gave warnings, the Persian-born al-Razi counseling against overuse, while the 10th century physician Ibn Wahshiyah warned of possible complications of hashish, even the possibility of death when mixed with other drugs. By the 13th century Islamic scientists published an entire book on the substance. Then, the danger of routine pot smoking to the public had become clearly evident. Simultaneously, the Spanish botanist Ibn al-Baytar published a description of its psychoactive properties, saying that it caused dementia in some users, the first known mention of such a connection.

The people of Central Asia, the Mongols, popularized the intoxicant. These fierce warriors were heavy users of alcohol and hashish, often using them together. It is held by some that the large-scale popularization of the intoxicant in the Middle East and North Africa was largely as a result of the Mongol invasions. As a result, the drug became widely popular in Syria and Egypt. This led to a lengthy period of cultural decadence, the so-called dark ages of the region, about 1250 to 1570 A.D., which is attributed to widespread use of hashish among the common people. Because of the corruption of society and reduced productivity, attempts were made to reverse the trend for addiction, which proved largely unsuccessful.

One reason for this attempted ban was the addiction of soldiers, in this case, those of Egypt's Mameluke dynasty, to the substance, a habit they acquired from interaction with the Mongols. Then, in the 13th century it was found that soldiers addicted to hashish were mentally and physically debilitated. Society's future was at stake. This is why various Islamic leaders attempted to correct this through destroying the intoxicating crops, confiscating ready-made material, and imposing taxes.

Yet, this was not a religious edict but, rather, one aimed at society at-large. After all, in tradition from the Greeks pioneering Islamic doctors used cannabis as a drug for a variety of conditions, including as a pain-killer and anesthetic. It was the respected legal scholar az-Zakarias who in the 14th century noted that the use of hashish would be lawful if consumed for "medical necessity to produce anesthesia for an amputation, and if consumed to still hunger," that is if the person wasn't inherently vulnerable to the addiction. This demonstrates the care inherent in Islamic civilization for its subjects.

Despite this, throughout much of the civilized world the main use was never for mere smoking. In medieval Europe hemp became a key crop for industrial purposes: rope, paper, textiles, sails, and more. In the 18th century it was listed as an important drug in various medical dispensaries, including those in the Americas. By 1776 Kentucky began growing the crop, while both George Washington and Thomas Jefferson grew it enthusiastically.

Upon being introduced by British physicians in the Americas cannabis quickly became an important drug. This expanded greatly through Victorian times up to the turn of the century. Then, recreational use and/or the smoking of the drug was virtually unknown.

The thriving, new society was in great need for medical therapies. No one was looking to cannabis to get high. In fact, by the 19th century it captured a strong position in Western medicine on a large scale. Regarding the British they accumulated their initial knowledge from India, where cannabis was widely used as a therapeutic. In 1839 an Irish physician at the Medical College of Calcutta, William B. O'Shaughnessy, published a detailed report on cannabis, which he called "Indian Hemp." Performing animal studies he determined that cannabis extracts were an effective means to treat a wide range of conditions, including epilepsy, an early Western proof regarding this disease. He also found it effective against rabies, joint pain, muscle aches, and chronic pain. In an 1860 report the Ohio Medical Society of Physicians proclaimed the drug effective against stomach pain, gastritis, psychosis, chronic cough, and neuralgia, actions now proven through the dispensing of today's CO_2 extract.

In the 1920s recreational use was popularized. This coincided with the plot to ban cannabis, including the industrial type. That ban was largely orchestrated by vested interests, such as the DuPont and Hearst families, which viewed it as a threat to their established interests, in this case the nylon and paper-milling industries, respectively. By 1942 it was removed from the US pharmacopoeia. This proved disastrous, as through this process the growing of all types of cannabis, including the highly valuable industrial type, was banned under threat of prosecution and imprisonment. The nutritional and industrial benefits of hemp were seemingly lost forever to the American people and the world at-large, largely as a consequence of the actions of a few criminal minds. So, too, was lost one of the most potent, effective natural cures known: the hemp-based phytochemicals, including the cannabinoids, simple terpenes, and the more complex terpenoid, Beta-caryophyllene.

Chapter Three

Recreational Use: a Panacea?

In antiquity there is recorded use of marijuana as a recreational drug. This occurred originally in the Indian subcontinent and also in Central Asia. More recently, it was popularized in 19th century Europe. As early as 1000 B.C. cannabis was used as an intoxicant in India and Iran. Later, it become popular in parts of the Middle East and Northern Africa, where it was known as hashish. It's popularity as a drug is a consequence of a novel capacity, which is its ability to alter the senses. What else could do what the drug could achieve? A person shortly after intake would experience a kind of elation, even euphoria. This was perhaps most vividly described by French poet Charles Baudelaire in his 19th century book *Les Paradis Artificiel*, that is 'Artificial Paradise.' Apparently, Baudelaire and associated French writers, such as Alexandre Dumas, didn't use mere cannabis but rather smoked a far more intoxicating type, the one with the resin concentrate, hashish. There can be no doubt that this type of marijuana is highly hallucinogenic. The authors became so consumed by their habit that they formed an infamous hashish circle, "Club des Hashischins." Let us see through an edited extract of the work, as described by J. Green in *Cannabis*, just what Baudelaire said about it, whether real or imagined:

> At first, a certain absurd, irresistible hilarity overcomes you. The most ordinary words, the simplest ideas, assume a new and bizarre aspect. This mirth (that is the sensation of amusement) is intolerable to you; but it is useless to resist. The demon has invaded you...
>
> It sometimes happens that people completely unsuited for word-play will improvise an endless string of puns and wholly improbable idea relationships fit to outdo the ablest masters of this preposterous craft. But after a few minutes the relation between ideas becomes so vague, and the thread of your thoughts grows so tenuous, that only your cohorts... can understand you.

He continues to explain the experience in detail:

> Next, your senses become extraordinarily keen and acute. Your sight is infinite. Your ear can discern the slightest perceptible sound, even through the shrillest of noises. The slightest ambiguities, the most inexplicable transpositions of ideas take place. In sounds there is color; in colors there is a music... You are sitting and smoking. You believe that you are sitting in your pipe, and that your pipe is smoking you. You are exhaling yourself in bluish clouds. This fantasy goes on for an eternity. A lucid interval, and a great expenditure of effort, permit you to look at the clock. The eternity turns out to have been only a minute.
>
> The third phase... is something beyond description. It is what the Orientals call 'kef' it is complete happiness. There is nothing whirling and tumultuous about it. It is a calm and placid beatitude. Every philosophical

problem is resolved. Every difficult question that presents a point of contention for theologians, and brings despair to thoughtful men, becomes clear and transparent. Every contradiction is reconciled. Man has surpassed the gods.

Ultimately, Baudelaire held hashish smoking in disregard, believing that the user would likely suffer psychological problems. "Morale" is the section of Baudelaire's remarks, where he says that while hashish certainly enhances the imagination and, thus, creativity, it is *highly dangerous to subordinate all such processes to the drug*. For creative artists to believe that they can create only when "high" is disastrous, he notes. Ultimately, 'cannabis destroys your personality and that was unacceptable.' This fact has commonly been confirmed in modern-day users.

His concluding remarks are as follows:

There, then, you are, for some hours yet, incapable of work, of action, and of energy. It is the punishment of an impious prodigality in which you have squandered your nervous force. You have dispersed your personality to the four winds of heaven—and now, what trouble to gather it up again and concentrate it!

Clearly, this is not a substance to take lightly or to use in a haphazard way. A person can readily become addicted to it. Too, of what real benefit is it to so dramatically alter the senses? It becomes clear, then, that recreational use has no major benefits and, rather, corrupts the user or at a minimum makes the person less efficient, if capable of clear and concise work at all. Frequently, in fact, the routine user becomes a virtual social invalid, as long as such a one is constantly smoking the drug.

By the middle of the 19th century the Club des Hashischins had broken up, but in strictly scientific terms it had done its work. In 1846 its instigator, Dr. Moreau, published his major work on cannabis, the 439-page book *De Hachish et de l'Alienation Mentale, Études Psychologiques* (Hashish and Mental Illness, Psychological Studies). Clearly, then, with the exception of rare cases, such as sufferers in chronic pain, cannabis smoking, or ingestion, cannot benefit the individual. As demonstrated by the Club members of old by no means can it achieve anything productive. In fact, it has the opposite effect, impeding productivity, let there be no mistake about it. Even so, like any addiction despite toxicity reactions people respond with denial.

Clearly, as a hallucinogen marijuana had a novel capacity for the people of that era, one not experienced with alcoholic beverages, the other heavily consumed intoxicant of the time. Yet, despite this, there are people all over the world, and surely numerous bloggers on the Internet, who insist that this is not the case and that marijuana is by no means toxic: to any degree. Even certain medical doctors make the claim that it possesses no danger and that at best that danger is minimal. As it turns out many of these medical doctors themselves are addicts. They often, though, change their views after attempting to purge themselves of the addiction.

Perhaps dangerous is not the proper word. Yet, to claim it is harmless is erroneous: and that is where the danger is. It should be respected for what it is: a potent medication. Moreover, it is bred to be an intoxicant by the privately operating marijuana growers themselves. These growers do this for financial gain, not for health advancement.

There are countless people who have gotten sick after smoking marijuana. Medicinal herbs simply don't do this, or if they do, it is exceedingly rare. In this regard it is not merely a matter of getting stoned. There are actual physical syndromes now being attributed exclusively to the drug's use. One such syndrome is known as "cannabinoid hyperemesis syndrome" or CHS. This even occurs in people who are seeking marijuana-based relief from nausea and vomiting. Who would have anticipated it? The fact is it is having the opposite effect, which is to trigger these two conditions. The symptoms of the syndrome include abdominal cramps, vicious, even projectile, vomiting, and a most unique symptom: the overwhelming urge for a hot shower. According to the testimonies of patients available online, this usually leads to numerous visits to the hospital. This results in CT scans, X-rays, and other useless procedures. All that is recorded is a healthy-appearing person who vomits a lot.

In 2004 a study was done on nine Australians identified with the syndrome. In seven instances "cessation of cannabis abuse led to cessation of the cyclical vomiting." There was no explanation for the most bizarre anomaly seen, which was the habit of taking scaldingly hot showers or baths, apparently to relieve their symptoms. Regardless, clearly this is a consequence of the over-excitation of neurological centers by the cannabis toxins.

The most thorough study to date on CHS was conducted in 2012 by D. A. Simonetto, who tested some 100 patients. He merely confirmed that for people who regularly smoke, nausea and vomiting are definite side effects, while a majority also experienced abdominal pain. Half the study participants mitigated their symptoms by bathing in scalding hot water. Said lead researcher Georgia Regents Medical Center's Larry Mellick, "Now, the treatment they were hoping would make them feel better is actually complicating their illness even more."

The illness is not uncommon, with some 200 case incidences in the U.S. reported. Despite this, as a rule physicians don't know about it," notes Dr. Larry Mellick. "It is not on everybody's radar just yet," he noted.

Consider the case of a patient who had been to the emergency room seven times before Mellick saw her, with several tests and scans that proved negative before she got the right diagnosis. This case, he says, is typical. "Every patient I've seen, here, has had multiple visits in ERs around...They've had CT scans, they've had lab tests, they've had ultrasounds. Repeatedly, nothing shows up. It's consistently negative, and the diagnosis just isn't being made." Obviously, then, marijuana is causing great corruption in users, confusing and scaring them, essentially creating a symptom-based paranoia.

Case reports often demonstrate toxicity never realized in research studies. Once again, certain Internet-related case histories are highly revealing. They paint a different picture from that issued by the marijuana apologists, those who claim that smoking is perfectly safe and that it in virtually all instances is non-toxic. Notice that smokers have formed a virtual global club, an entity unto themselves, with their own social norms, even their own language. Speaking in code, they have become a unit of apologists for their habit, much like alcoholics living outside of reality. These anonymous case histories, edited for readability, are as follows:

I started smoking pot when I was 12 years old. As I got into my teens, 13 through 15, the availability of better quality product became the norm. Generally, we're talking 1985, 1986 time frame. During that time actual green bud was extremely rare to find. Hash was found everywhere and that was what we were smoking 99% of the time. From 12 years old to 15 years old I was a happy little stoner. One day some friends and myself were having a session. We rolled out a 7 gram chimney. Rolled it into a tube, stuck a pin through 1 end and lit the other end. In 20 minutes three of us smoked the entire joint. Needless to say we were ripped.

At this point the man is clearly hallucinating and has taken himself out of normal, real perceptions: purposely so:

I was sitting on the couch, zoning out on a spec on the white drywall when I began to get the spins, and I felt a ball in my throat that *did not make me feel well.* I tried to maintain, but it became overwhelming to the point where I had to get up off the couch. I went to the bathroom and turned the water on and pressed my forehead to the cold spout and splashed water on my face.

The sickness was all over me. It was so incredibly unpleasant I cannot begin to describe to you the horror of it. I threw up violently, then sat down on the toilet and exploded out that end as well. I turned the light off. It was pitch black in the bathroom. Trying to do anything to escape the terrible sickness I was experiencing, I began to hallucinate, seeing colorful patterns amidst the darkness. Nothing I did made me feel better. Cleaning myself up best I could, I got the (expletive deleted) out of there and left my friend's house without saying goodbye. Walking down the street, I was watching the pavement as it passed under my feet. The crisp, cold, damp air in the night coupled with me concentrating on watching the pavement as I walked was the only thing that allowed me any relief or ability to maintain. I walked, and walked, and walked some more. In total I walked roughly 3 hours. I finally walked home and hit my bed and passed out.

Is it not incredible? It reads like a novel, yet it is a true example, on the ground, of the actions of this hallucinogen. He continued:

> Some might say this was an isolated incident and that maybe I had a stomach bug or a bad piece of meat or something, no. I tried smoking pot again after that, and every time I tried there after, the same crippling sickness crawled up on me. So, by age 15, I stopped smoking pot. I tried years later here and there, and the same reaction would befall me.

In response a poster said:

> Something like this happened to me just last night. Not a regular smoker (using it) just 3 or 4 times a year, last night I was having panic attacks, so I thought it would be a good way to chill out. So I got some from my brother, who bought it from some guy he knows; I smoked two bowls and about an hour later I smoked a blunt. After about 10 minutes I was dripping in sweat. I went through an entire roll of paper towels wiping myself off. I couldnt feel if I was hot or cold. All I could feel was pulsating in my body. Running to the bathroom I threw up and peed all over myself in the process. This happened twice. I ended up passing out on the bathroom floor because it was cold and felt good, even though I was laying in a pool of my own sweat. Waking up after I don't know how long, I was still sweating but not nearly as bad. I was so cold from being on that bathroom floor...I thought I was going to die on that bathroom floor.

Yet another poster chimed in about a similar experience, once again claiming that the frightening, bizarre reaction led to his quitting:

Oh, man, I had a bad trip, too. I was throbbing and couldn't breathe. I thought if I took a big enough breath my heart would explode. Eventually, I threw up after getting my limbs back from the heaviness. That was the first and last time I will EVER smoke.

The real world of smokers is best revealed by such experiences. A poster added that for many the temperature regulation issue is common, with his experiencing, alternatively, "freezing, burning, and sweating." Once, he added, he had insomnia as a consequence, *lying awake for 28 hours*, hallucinating at the same time.

The addictive nature of the drug is clearly evident by such experiences. Noted a man who had smoked for some 20 years:

I smoked at least once a day, up to 4 joints a day by myself. I stopped smoking a week ago, but I am completely miserable. I'm always dreaming of using, sometimes when I am desperate, waking up in sweats, searching the entire house for a roach.

This was responded to by another user, as follows:

It's been two weeks since I vaporized my last bowl. Since then, I've gotten so desperate I've been smoking resin. Last night, I used rubbing alcohol to get the resin out of my bong, smoking it after the alcohol evaporated. It tasted awful and barely got me high, but tonight I did it again, and I was so impatient that I put the resin-alcohol solution in the oven to help it evaporate. This is how desperate I've become —I've risked burning down my house in order to get marginally high.

Why would anyone want to put themselves and/or their family through this? It gives an internal window to the nature of not merely marijuana addiction but all other habituations:

> After using heavily for the past seven years and basically all day every day for the last 6 months my side effects are major. I still can't sleep properly, although at least now I'm getting six hours, though there is nausea daily. I'm suffering hot and cold sweats and am freezing, right now, while a half hour ago I was boiling.
> I haven't eaten properly since I stopped. What I don't like is that I feel spaced out constantly...I feel like I'm bent even when I'm not and not bent in a calm, relaxing way, either.

At this point an investigator weighs in. The entire thread becomes highly revealing for the sake of all those who are partaking in the addiction. It demonstrates that much of the apologetics for the substance arises from users themselves:

> I am a researcher at a university and have studied the effects of drugs, particularly alcohol, on the brain for the past decade or so. Like many of my friends and colleagues, I consider marijuana to be a relatively low-risk drug when used in moderation by responsible adults. However, I am now forced to admit that my view of the discontinuation syndrome was naive and that I was completely unprepared for it myself:
>
> Week 1: Despite missing my evening smoking session and feeling some mild irritability, I felt fine.
>
> Week 2: Mild flu-like symptoms, which I assumed to be viral in nature though it did not exactly feel viral. No real desire to smoke marijuana. I assumed I was out of the woods and had gotten off easy.

Week 3: Sudden onset of incredibly intense and vivid dreams. Profuse sweating at night. Difficulty discerning dreaming from waking state. Lack of energy. Upset stomach. Absolutely no appetite. Unable to focus. Saw my primary care physician. All labs normal.

Week 4: This is where the real problems began for me. Sudden onset of intense, full body anxiety.... This led to complete insomnia for days. A very deep feeling of dread and a sense that I was going completely insane. Crying spells that came from nowhere....

Week 5: The intense anxiety slowly began to dissipate... was able to sleep for four to six hours a night, which is approaching normal for me. Appetite slowly came back but the thought of eating was unpleasant. Feeling of confidence began to return. Feelings of hopelessness and of going crazy began to diminish.

He continued:

The cravings have pretty much subsided but not completely. When I get bored is when it is the strongest. I have experienced the sweating, *severe diarrhea, migraine headaches and sleeplessness....* I have *hidden this addiction from family for so long and it's nice to not have to worry if someone is going to stop by and smell it and catch me.*

There is no reason to live in such a way. For those seeking pain relief or other benefits extracts of the industrial type will suffice. Once again, the benefits of recreational marijuana smoking are outweighed by the drawbacks.

In cases of cannabinoid hyperemesis syndrome, that is the uncontrollable vomiting, doctors theorize that the active ingredient in marijuana, THC, overwhelms the body's autonomic nervous system. This is obviously the case, since it is also this system which is involved in temperature regulation. There is also nausea, once again as a result of autonomic nervous system overload. That leads to a condition similar to the morning sickness of pregnancy.

These are extreme reactions, far more so than those seen with other addictive dietary agents such as chocolate and caffeine.

One of the more neglected side-effects of the drug is relaxation, excessively so. Yet another is sleepiness. Still another is heaviness, that is heaviness of the body and limbs. There is also a sense of apathy. All these are noxious. They cause a state of non-productivity. How can the person achieve even a reasonable level of productivity when burdened with such symptomology? It demonstrates the nature of an intoxicant, proving that such a substance cannot benefit people to any degree and, ultimately, always interferes with their potential.

To a lesser degree the same is surely true of dietary substances. At the turn of the century books for common people were published warning about the danger of stimulants, especially for the chronically ill. These stimulants for which warnings were issued included black coffee, black tea, refined sugar, and chocolate or cocoa. Consider the latter. Because of its powerful mood-altering agents, the theobromines, chocolate, too, can be addictive. Excess consumption can in some individuals cause considerable irritability to the nervous system. It may also agitate the adrenal glands, causing them to be depleted. In some cases constant, daily use is associated with outright disease such as the onset of anxiety-neurosis, depression, chronic fatigue syndrome, and tuberculosis.

Yet, the primary subject, here, is marijuana. Like cocoa, despite the addictive potential it is a food. With cocoa or chocolate the form does matter. Extensively heat-treated material, combined with heat-treated milk and refined sugar, is more noxious than the minimally processed type, also the types which are lower in sugar. Marijuana is the same, since it is primarily the heat-exposed type, that is the smoked material, that has the strongest addictive powers. Heat causes a dramatic increase in the primary addictive chemical, tetrahydrocannabinol. In contrast, if a person ate the raw, fresh leaves, there would be far less likelihood of addictive consequences, although the consumption of the flowering tops or resinous buds is addictive. Yet, even in the bred marijuana, in the raw plant leaves, that is the juiced plant matter, there is little to none of this psychoactive chemical found.

To avoid the psychoactive form of hemp is easy. A person merely never consumes the type bred for psychoactive properties. Instead, the individual only uses so-called industrial hemp, preferably that grown without chemicals or poisons. The key word is consume rather than smoke.

Even the smoke from burning brush fires is unhealthy and can quickly overwhelm a person. So is that which issues from the burning of coal. All such smoke is irritating to lungs and cardiovascular system.

Is marijuana the worst, most dangerous drug in the world? Of course it is not. Yet, this has nothing to do with its addictive, hallucinogenic properties. A hallucinogen is a substance or molecular complex which alters sensations of reality, that is causes hallucinations. Moreover, hallucinations are "profound distortions in perceptions." Who wants to undergo such a reaction, where such a one doesn't even know what is going on about him? Under its influence people see images, hear sounds, and feel sensations that appear to be real but are not. In some cases the intake of hallucinogens leads to rapid, intense emotional swings.

Yet, it is said that there is no possible toxicity with cannabis, some authors claiming that statements otherwise are mere "propaganda..." There are actually people throughout the alternative media, for instance, the Internet, claiming that the smoking or ingestion of marijuana is "perfectly safe... Yet, even in the commonly consumed foods of this earth and its herbs virtually nothing is "perfectly safe," especially various plant complexes with mood-altering and hallucinogenic actions.

There is clearly a bias in the marijuana legalization movement in regard to its consumption. Moreover, as has been demonstrated, here, there are countless people, smokers, who are seemingly in a state of denial. Yet, they are waking up to this, often determining on their own that the smoking of hallucinogenic marijuana is not a good idea. The purpose, here, is to outline any real dangers of marijuana smoking without bias, while also demonstrating any potential benefits.

That bias or, in fact, scheming against all things hemp is very real. Is it not bizarre? There are other plants which are drug-like which also have both positive and negative aspects, opium poppies being an example. Poppy seeds are highly nutritious, just as are the seeds of the marijuana plant, known as hemp seeds. Yet, the drug extracts of the plant, opiates, are highly destructive and addictive. Even so, opiates have decided value as pain-killing agents, codeine and morphine being prominent examples. Too, the coca leaf has some minor health benefits, although its refined concentrates, cocaine and heroin, are among the most addictive, physiologically corrupting drugs known. Yet, it makes no sense at all. It is illegal to grow non-hallucinogenic hemp in the United States. For those who wish to consume hemp seeds, the seed oil, or the protein it has to be imported from other countries.

Yet, this issue of the harmlessness of drug-like marijuana is a curious element. It is often stated that regarding marijuana its toxicity is not an issue, since, compared to highly potent illicit drugs, such as heroin and opium, it is a minor player. This is mere rationalization. No hallucinogenic, addictive drug is a "minor issue." All of them have a degree of toxicity, leading to damaging effects upon the human body as well as the overall psychological state. A lesser effect is not necessarily 'better.' Even so, through such rationalization, it is held, marijuana can be consumed with relative impunity. This is the danger in it. In other words, its potential for causing human damage is disregarded by users and their apologists.

Furthermore, there is the issue of the use of addictive material, "medically." No doubt, because of its actions on the nerve centers there is some value in it. After all, it does numb pain, especially so-called neuropathic pain. In patients with multiple sclerosis, for instance, it has been determined that "smoked cannabis" is superior to "placebo in reducing spasticity and pain" and even offers aid "beyond currently prescribed medications." Such use should be fully allowed, legally: especially under dispensation by a physician. Yet, still, there remains that ever-present danger of addiction development. For multiple sclerosis and/or neuropathic pain patients it is superior to use the CO_2 extract. The results will be more profound, without the risk of habituation. Because of its dense supply of Beta-caryophyllene it will prove to be highly effective in pain relief and also the purging of inflammation, and this type can be taken internally and applied topically. Plus, long term, the smoking of any substance is pro-inflammatory.

Chapter Four

Hormones, Sexual Organs, and More

The hormonal apparatus is heavily under the control of the nervous system. For instance, it is the nerve centers, the hypothalmus and the pituitary, as well as the pineal gland, which are the ultimate controlling agents of the hormone system.

Also known as the endocrine system these glands are essentially condensations of nerve tissue. Thus, any imbalance in brain and/or nerve function affects them, including imbalances in the endocannabinoid system. Just like the cannabinoids in marijuana the brain's endocannabinoid molecules exert significant powers over memory, mood, appetite, and the regulation of responses to pain as well as inflammation. All these elements are ultimately interconnected with endocrine function.

The endocannabinoid and endocrine systems act as a team in order to keep the body in balance. In fact, the cannabinoids act as key activators or regulators of hormone gland function. Cannabinoid receptors are found in virtually all glands. In this regard the cannabinoid receptor complex is essential for a most crucial issue, which is the maintenance of optimal function of the human organ system, a phenomenon known as homeostasis.

Homeostasis means balance. This is the balance necessary for the body to adapt to stress and/or toxicity: for it to maintain optimal function. There is a most profound example of this within human physiology, which is a process mentioned previously known as *autophagy*. This involves the normal actions of human cells, in this case to eliminate their own corrupt matter. All cells must process waste matter to be either digested and eliminated or recycled. This is essential to life itself. In fact, cells which are able to efficiently process wastes or excesses, as well as to recycle any potentially constructive elements, live longer than cells with impaired capacities to do so. In some studies when artificially supported cells are able to routinely purge their wastes, they live indefinitely. The combined efforts of the endocrine secretions, along with endocannabinoids, is essential for assisting cells in waste removal and recycling and also in the efficient rebuilding of aging cells.

The endocrine centers: toxicity of marijuana smoke

There is no means for the endocrine system to handle the toxicity of plant smoke. Nor can they handle a constant overload of the highly addictive compound THC. The cannabinoid receptors themselves are a fixed component of human cells, being embedded within the cell membranes, including those of hormone gland cells. It is a highly sophisticated system, one that should not be overwhelmed or corrupted to any degree. Stress surely overwhelms it. So does the consumption of noxious substances, particularly alcohol and illicit drugs. Prescription drugs also disrupt this system, often massively so. So do residues of pesticides, herbicides, and fungicides. All such toxins cause the endocannabinoid system to go into overload, ultimately depleting it.

Pot smoking also does precisely this but in a novel way. This is by causing this system to be overwhelmed by specific cannabinoids, leading, essentially, to a cannabinoid imbalance. One group of cannabinoid receptor sites is overloaded to the detriment of another. The circuits in one realm are fully hyper-excited, leading to physiological imbalances. To a degree all potent, neurologically active drugs operate in this manner. This can be highly destructive, since the virtual control centers of life itself, the brain and its substructures, can be adversely affected. The greatest offenders of this neurological overload are alcoholic beverages, with high-THC marijuana coming a close second.

No one should take self-intoxication lightly. This is a low ebb for humanity. There is no known overall benefit of such intoxication. People lose control of their senses. Often, they make fools of themselves. In the extreme they place themselves and others in danger. How can there be any benefit to this?

The endocrine glands in particular are highly vulnerable to the noxious effects of intoxicants. This includes that all-important master gland of the hormone system, the hypothalamus. Like other brain organs it is heavily vested with cannabinoid receptors. In a 1984 article in *NIDA Research Monograph* it was shown that standard, crude marijuana, that is pot, as well as the key active ingredient,

THC, have powerful, in fact, overwhelming actions on the hypothalamus, causing a suppression of three key sex and/or reproductive hormones. These hormones are FSH and LH as well as prolactin. These are crucial pre-hormones for stimulating the various gonadal glands, including the ovaries and testes. Yet, these hormones also act upon the adrenal glands, yet another producer of sex steroids.

Suppression or blockage of normal sex hormone production is highly unhealthy, especially in developing youths as well as in pregnant and lactating females. The study, done in primates, determined that high-THC marijuana intake causes decreases in the hypothalamic-pituitary hormones to such a degree that ovulation and sperm production were negatively affected. In the lab animal toxicity was observed in the ovaries and testes. Too, it is speculated that the ovum may be damaged as a result of exposure to THC, leading to the observed retardation of fetal growth. Even so, many of the disturbances in hormone status were reversed upon cessation of exposure. In contrast, oftentimes such damage by alcohol is not so forgiving.

It has always been speculated that pot negatively affects manhood, with even some reports, difficult to substantiate, claiming that it causes shrinkage of male sex organs. Even so, as mentioned previously marijuana smoke causes direct toxicity to testosterone and its trophic pituitary hormone, LSH. In smokers levels of testosterone dropped significantly, nearly 50%, while LSH declined some 15%. Moreover, the smoke was found to consume key antioxidants, notably glutathione peroxidase and antioxidants in general. This was thought to be due to the noxious effects of nitric oxide, levels of which are dramatically elevated as a result of ingestion of the smoke: up to 200% above controls.

Thyroid and adrenals

By no means is the smoking of any substance beneficial to these key endocrine glands. That's because the thyroid and adrenal glands react to inhaled smoke as a toxin. This forces them to overwork in order to purge the body of smoke's toxic metabolites. Furthermore, THC has direct toxicity to the thyroid organ, blocking the production of active thyroid hormone. This blockade leads to heaviness of the limbs, fatigue, and exhaustion. It also may lead to cardiac arrhythmias, even in some more rare cases, heart attacks. The adrenals suffer the consequences, too, as they are highly sensitive to inhaled carbon dioxide and carbon monoxide.

The unborn: stillbirths and more

It is clearly apparent that the regular smoking of any substance, including plant matter from tobacco and marijuana, is dangerous to the developing fetus. By no means is it safe to any degree for a pregnant woman to smoke these drugs. Regarding the inhalation of cannabis smoke this was confirmed by work published in the *Obstetrics and Gynecology*, the study surveying the relationship between stillbirth and a range of different drug-related risk factors. The use of marijuana, it was determined significantly elevated the risk for fetal mortality. "When [the results are] controlled for cigarette smoking, marijuana use is [still] associated with an increased risk of stillbirth," lead researcher Dr. Michael Varner said. "Because marijuana use may be increasing with increased legalization, the relevance of these findings may increase as well."

Some 663 stillbirths between March 2006 and September 2008 were evaluated. Here, umbilical cord blood samples were tested as well as maternal blood. This was then compared to the values from some 1900 live births. Nearly 95% of the stillbirths, Varner found, were associated with some type of substance abuse, with marijuana being the number one culprit. The other major factor was cigarette smoking and also exposure to second-hand smoke. Without doubt, it was determined, there is an association between marijuana smoking and deaths of fetuses.

What happens when a pregnant woman smokes marijuana? The drug crosses the placenta to the baby. Marijuana, like cigarette smoke, contains toxins that keep the developing infant from getting the proper supply of oxygen it needs to grow. Regardless, realizing the action of pot on humans no one could consider smoking this drug to be safe and/or healthy for the developing fetus.

Consider the following case report based on personal, direct contact:

> CASE HISTORY: A pregnant woman smoked pot for several months during her pregnancy. At nearly the 8th month she had a stillbirth. Autopsy confirmed that chemicals from marijuana smoke were the cause. What was discovered was the baby stopped developing at ten weeks due to oxygen deprivation.

It makes sense. Smoking marijuana increases the levels of carbon monoxide and carbon dioxide in the blood, which reduce the oxygen supply to the baby. Smoking the drug during pregnancy can increase the risk of miscarriage, low birth-weight, premature births, developmental delays, and behavioral as well as learning disabilities. Studies have shown that children who were exposed to marijuana during pregnancy sometimes have problems focusing their attention and solving problems. Children of heavy pot users may also develop problems with short-term memory, concentration, and judgment. In fetal development it is not nearly as dangerous as alcohol, but it is still noxious, and in the cause of stillbirths it may be just as dangerous. Yet, can anyone imagine it, that is the combined effect upon the fetus from drinking alcohol *and* smoking pot?

Chemical imbalances caused by pot

There are a number of imbalances which occur in the body as a result of pot smoking. Marijuana raises the levels of pro-inflammatory hormones, the prostaglandins of the E-2 series, that is PGE2. This readily induces inflammation in the cardiac arteries and the arteries of the brain, constricting blood flow to these organs. Narrowed arteries require a higher degree of blood pressure to pump the blood through, explaining the consistent moderate-to-mild rise in blood pressure seen in users. PGE2 can also cause inflammation in the blood-brain barrier, weakening it, allowing the marijuana chemicals more ready access.

Significant amounts of the highly potent neurologically active agent, THC, may now enter. This may result in not only hypertension and cardiac arrhythmia but also migraine headaches, dull, aching headaches, blurry vision, sleeping disorders, ringing of the ears, joint inflammation, and also liver/kidney disorders. With aggressive use the drug could cause heart attacks and brain hemorrhage, that is vascular stroke, leading to brain tissue death. PGE2 is widely recognized as an unhealthy metabolite. Constant pot smoking keeps the levels dangerously high.

No doubt, the body recognizes the various chemicals from marijuana smoke as noxious, in fact, as toxins. These toxins directly poison healthy cells. Exposure to these chemicals on a consistent basis leads to a constant state of chemical toxicity. This, then, deadens the cells' functions, particularly the functional capacity of the nerve cells. For the repeat offender it's a constant assault, and the body has great difficulty recovering from it.

Marijuana so greatly upsets the nerves that it can lead to sexual exhaustion. This is a result of a numbing effect on the nervous system component, the parasympathetic element, which is responsible for sustaining erection during sex. Ultimately, the marijuana chemicals overtake the acetylcholine. This leads to suppression also of nitric acid and cyclic GMP. All this impedes male potency to the extreme.

Once pot's chemicals corrupt the nervous system, it is difficult to restore balance. Essentially, at this point the psychoactive chemicals "numb" the nerve endings. Unless this is corrected there is the potential for permanent impotence. The capacity for orgasm is also completely corrupted. Psychoactive components of marijuana fully deplete the key neurotransmitters needed for normal sexual function.

The attack on the male sex glands is thorough. The production of seminal fluid collapses, while the function of the testes, in general, is impeded. There is less and less ejaculation matter. Ultimately, seminal and testicular secretions halt, that is dry up. At that point permanent impotence may set in.

In addition, there is measurable liver damage in users. In marijuana smokers, the GGT activity was nearly 90%

higher than that of the control group, while SGPT levels were elevated some 20%. Compared to non-smokers alkaline phosphatase was up some 120%. In addition, the bilirubin level, a marker of liver cell damage, rose 40%. Combined with the liver enzyme abnormalities this is a sign of stress on this organ of detoxification as it attempts to purge toxins in the smoke. The levels of a key neurotransmitter processing enzyme, acetyl cholinesterase, were nearly 12% lower than controls.

Just what causes an addiction to pot has not been fully established. Some people, it must be noted, readily become habituated, while others do not. Ultimately, marijuana causes a reduction in the number of CB1 receptors in the brain. This may explain the increasing dependence on the substance to gain the desired effect. As reported in *Molecular Psychiatry*, 2012, after a month of abstinence, the receptor levels returned to normal, the exception being in the section known as the hippocampus, the arena where memory is formed. There is surely alteration in the production of neurotransmitters, largely mediated by the increase in nitric oxide levels. Depletion of such substances leads to a dependence and the need to consume increasing amounts to gain the desired effect.

These alterations largely explain the addiction as well as the complexity of withdrawals. Some people can merely quit outright, while others struggle with it. Even so, unlike withdrawal from heavy alcohol or cocaine use marijuana withdrawal is virtually never lethal, although suicide has been reported in people who are unsuccessful in such withdrawal. In contrast, alcohol withdrawal is often a medical emergency. Without significant therapeutic intervention, it can prove deadly.

Even so, it is understood why people turn to pot. Often, it is the same people who also turn to alcohol. It is commonly those who suffer psychological problems. Life itself for many smokers seems "empty." Perhaps its an issue of hidden anger or possibly frustration. It may also be related to the way the person is raised. In the case of young men possibly it is related to an oppressive father. Clearly, in many instances there is a rebellion aspect. Pot smokers have hidden or repressed anger. They use the drug to mellow out.

Rather than increasing productivity pot smoking reduces it. This is in part a consequence of the action of THC on the neuromuscular system. Yet, no one would purposely seek to cause self-harm. People are users because in some manner their bodies are deficient: socially, emotionally, and spiritually. It may be a consequence of nutritional deficiencies and, thus, defects in brain metabolism itself. Here, a person suffers from a racing mind and uses cannabis for sedation. There may also be self-doubt, even low self-confidence. Pot smoking suppresses this through the much-desired temporary euphoria.

Pot smokers are also commonly addicted to sugar and chocolate. Both these 'foods' cause temporary sensations of elation.

Yet, this is by no means an attempt to excuse the use. The same could be said for the taker of alcohol. Both substances cause a temporary boost in mood. If a person is unable to relax, there are other ways to deal with this, including the intake of herbal teas and also the consumption of B vitamins as well as the regular consumption of the caryophyllene-rich wild oregano-hemp complex.

Besides, it must be asked, "Why is the system so upset that a person cannot relax? Is it in part due to a lack of belief in anything supernatural? The heart-felt belief in a supreme Being creates peace within the heart, and people can readily find solace in this. For instance, says the grand, sophisticated Qur'aan, the holy book of the Islamic faith, human "hearts find peace" in the remembrance of God. It's how the heart is made to thrive. Turning all stresses and sources of hurt and emotional distress over to God is therapeutic. The thoughtful thinking of and consideration of this almighty One always creates a sense of softness and inner peace. Too, He is considerate of us, with all that He has provided. Why wouldn't human beings be considerate in response?

It is surely a key part of the answer. Clearly, there is great peace in prayer. Rather than a public display, which, in fact, can be irritating this is the prayer within the heart of a person, in peace and solace, privately. It is exclusively between the individual and the almighty creator. Despite this, there are people who have extreme imbalances within their nervous systems and despite attempts at prayer and meditation readily descend into nervousness or nervous agitation. While prayer will help they still need a 'chemical treatment' to create a deeper, more consistent sense of balance. They attempt to use prayer or invocations, for instance, at night to sleep. Yet, despite this, their minds still race and sleeping or relaxation is difficult. Clearly, such people are deficient in cannabinoids. Thus, the intake of this complex, along with heart-felt worship and prayer—in the peace of a person's own heart—is a powerful formula for the elimination of nervous agitation.

Prayer even helps a person fall asleep, especially if it is combined with cannabinoid therapy. It also helps a person relax when stricken with grief or overcome by frustration or anger. So, do use the prayer in any way that is effective but also support this with cannabinoid therapy.

Chapter Five

Marijuana, Good and Bad

People who smoke marijuana should be aware of the acute, toxic effects as well as any chronic toxicity. There are many smokers who seemingly have no obvious effects, while there are still others who readily develop the typical reactions. It may have to do with the physiological reserve of the individual. For instance, there are people who are of strong stock versus those who are rather frail. The frail type of people typically have insufficiency in adrenal function. Such weak adrenal people are highly vulnerable to intoxicants and/or stimulants. People with fine hair and who are blond and blue-eyed will also find themselves more readily intoxicated by the substance. As well, those who are on psychotropic drugs or who regularly drink alcohol are more likely to be reactive than those who merely smoke pot alone.

In many individuals smoking marijuana results in predictable signs and symptoms. Upon eating it, that is the hallucinogenic grade, those symptoms may also occur but often to a lesser degree. These reactions and side effects include:

- dryness of the mouth
- impaired short-term memory
- impaired perception
- disruption in appetite
- impaired motor skills
- redness of the eyes
- inability to cope with reality
- laziness
- apathy

These consequence are not as dire as those seen with the more noxious addictive substances, such as cocaine, heroin, and alcohol, but they are still significant. Yet, it is disconcerting that individuals suffer memory issues and impaired perception as well as a distortion in their coping ability. More significant, deleterious effects, which are more rarely seen, include the following:

- panic attacks
- sense of internal panic
- acute psychosis
- paranoia
- suicidal thoughts

It's CB1 that is the issue

In the manifestation of side effects, no doubt, CB1 receptors play a crucial role. Found mainly in the brain and spinal cord these receptors are so common in the central nervous system that they are known as "brain cannabinoid receptors." In contrast, CB2 sites are known as "peripheral cannabinoid receptors." CB1 is found in a particularly high density in the most primitive centers of the brain, the ones that control involuntary actions, like the hippocampus, basal ganglia, and cerebellum. In contrast, CB2 receptors are most densely placed in organs such as the testes, ovaries, liver, and spleen as well as white blood cells, where CB1 receptors are not typically seen.

The receptors exist in order to receive not only dietary cannabinoids but also those that are made within the body: the endocannabinoids. One issue is certain. Whether from the diet or produced within the human tissues the cannabinoids have a profound influence on the function of the internal organs, most dramatically on the brain and other nerve tissues. They act as regulatory complexes which aid in neurotransmitter synthesis and in the control of cell function. It is a sophisticated balancing act which is performed at the cellular level.

For optimal health it is crucial to consume cannabinoids and also to aid the body in the synthesis of the internal ones. There is yet another key to such health. This is the maintenance in the health and status of the receptor sites, whether CB1 or CB2. It has now been discovered that in many diseases there is a decline in the quantity of these receptors, for instance, the reduction in CB1 receptors in Huntington's disease. In addition, in schizophrenia a deficiency in cannabinoid receptors has been reported, where the brain has a high demand due to the deficiency for binding cannabinoids. In other words, it is working hard to utilize them and, thus, concentrates, for instance, the naturally occurring ones: some twice the level of normal.

While CB1 activation has its pros and cons the potential for side effects and toxicity must be reviewed. No one can say that marijuana is entirely safe. It can be said that in comparison it is less destructive to the body than hard drugs, like alcohol and cocaine. Yet, when it comes to human health, there is no room in medicine for false information. Nor is there any allowance for mere hype. The medicating of an individual is a serious issue. It should be based on factual information. This is the approach that will be taken regarding medical marijuana as well as the recreational drug itself.

There's an implied view that it is just weed, so what's the big deal? Why not smoke it? It's just an herb. The question is can marijuana be regarded as entirely safe for everyone and anyone without serious side effects, as some proponents claim: as certain medical authors even proclaim? Is it really safe to smoke, regularly, any plant matter without major risk of toxicity?

Here, it is suggested that marijuana not be smoked, especially regularly. Nor should it be consumed regularly. Why do so? This high-THC plant has been purposely altered in order to cause people to become addicted. Plus, heating dramatically increases the THC content. Then, this substance acts as an intoxicant, causing a major change in mood and awareness to such a degree that, often, users don't even know who they are or where they are. How can that be natural?

Man-made or, more correctly, man-altered marijuana is no longer an herb but is instead a drug. This is particularly true of the dried, flowering plant. The most potent type is that harvested when the flower turns to buds, where the hallucinogenic resin forms. Regarding this type of cannabis it acts as a drug whether smoked or consumed.

Then, since it is potent why do people use it? It is not for nutritional purposes or as a rule for the treatment of disease. The majority of people use it, because of its mood-altering properties, that is they take it to get high, that is they use it to dramatically alter their mood sensations in the brain, in other words, to become intoxicated.

The same is true of alcohol. Both are readily available and can be consumed without any obvious destructive effects: at least in the early phases. This does not, though, mean that they are safe long-term.

Intoxicants may be described as substances which create the propensity for being abused. They are addictive and may overwhelm the unsuspecting user. In this regard they create temporary sensations that appear beneficial while upon elimination after prolonged use lead to withdrawal symptoms. They are also substances which, after withdrawal, may leave residual effects.

Those who argue that there are more noxious intoxicants and addictive agents than marijuana are correct. Yet, this does not absolve it from the potential of causing toxicity, whether long-term or short-term.

Provable reports and research demonstrating such toxicity must be reviewed. To refuse to do so is no different than drug companies corrupting their own research to disguise side effects. Monsanto, Eli Lilly, G.D. Searle, and Merck have all done so. Marijuana must be analyzed for what it is: good and bad.

First, though, what is this 'bad?' It relates to the fact that smoking marijuana corrupts the thinking process. Regardless, why would anyone want to become intoxicated? Why subject the body to such a state? Why cause it to endure the potential for harm? Isn't life itself sufficiently satisfying to exist without any such a substance-induced state? Cannot a person become high on life itself?

Even so, there is the good, the positive benefits of marijuana. It has pain-numbing actions, along with certain anti-cancer powers. It is a muscle relaxant—the smoked kind, the drug. Yet, as will be demonstrated, here, the negatives outweigh the positives largely because of its addictive nature and the degree of addiction it causes.

So, it is clear. Of the millions of users in the United States alone relatively few use it for anything other than a drug, in lay terms, to get "stoned." Then, this is often in total disregard to its addictive effects and/or toxicity. Thus, it is necessary to outline any real dangers of marijuana smoking without bias, while also listing any benefits.

There is denial in regard to all addictive substances. This includes food-like drugs such as refined sugar. It does no good to live in such a denial. The person may end up contracting diabetes, even heart disease: even having a stroke and/or heart attack, all because of lying to the self. Other such addictive substances include caffeine and, therefore, coffee as well as cola bean and, therefore, soft drinks. All lead to a degree of withdrawal symptoms upon complete elimination from the diet.

Regarding marijuana, it is the flowering tops in particular and also the leaves that can be potentially addictive. This is primarily a result of heat exposure. As mentioned previously heat causes a dramatic increase in the main addictive chemical, tetrahydrocannabinol (THC).

Interestingly, in the raw plant, that is the juiced plant matter, the psychoactive chemical is not an issue. Nor is it found to any major degree in the cold-pressed seed oil, or, if it is found, it is in minor amounts. As well, the flowering tops contain the densest amount of the hallucinogen THC and its precursors.

Some hallucinogens are more dangerous than others. Marijuana is said to be one of the least dangerous of these. Yet, this is not entirely true. Though rare, in some people the drug can lead to attempted suicide and even the act itself.

So, today, the hallucinogenic type is consumed without warning. It is found as the dried plant, either leaves or buds or both. Or, it can be found as a pellet, which is concentrated resin. Commonly, it is mixed with tobacco and smoked. The dried herb itself may be hand-rolled in paper and smoked like a cigarette, called a "joint."

The burning of the plant causes corruption in the molecular structure, and as a result rather non-toxic compounds are turned into potentially noxious ones, particlarly THC. After inhaling the smoke the THC is quickly absorbed, directly into the bloodstream. From there it is carried to the brain, where it exhibits intensive effects. It's supposed to help depression, anxiety, and a sense of gloom. Yet, in many cases it worsens these states.

In contrast, the other type of cannabis, the so-called industrial hemp, is free of any such psychoactive properties, as well as any propensity for addiction. This is in relation to the hemp plant, the industrial hemp: the one used for the making of rope, paper, and other matter. With this type of marijuana there are no risks. From it is made even food-like products: hemp seed protein and hemp seed oil. Additionally, this is the source of the special kind of plant concentrate, a medicinal substance described previously: the CO_2 extract.

With pot, there is a considerable difference in the interactions. Upon the consumption of THC, either as smoke or edibles, a wave of this compound flows into the brain. There, it attaches to cannabinoid receptors, the CB1 type. These receptors are a natural component to brain tissue, basically coating vast areas of this organ. These receivers of THC are found in highest concentration in the thinking part of the brain, the cortex. The receptors are also found in dense amounts in the hypothalmus, the arena responsible for the control over the endocrine system, including those regions involved in appetite control. There is also a high density in the basal ganglia, the region in the brain that controls involuntary movements. The hippocampus, too, is CB1 receptor-rich, and this brain component controls memory function.

The existence of these receptors in these sites largely explains marijuana's effects, alteration in the basic thinking processes, appetite, and muscular processes.

Brain damage and self-destruction

While marijuana is not nearly as deadly as other 'illicit' drugs and alcohol, or even prescription drugs, for that matter, there are some clear downsides. Consider the issue of memory, that is the ability to hold pieces of information in mind. This is diminished in long-term marijuana smokers. There is also as described in the *Journal of the American Heart Association* a link to heart disorders, particularly in young users. Additionally, as demonstrated in a 2012 article in the *British Medical Journal,* cannabis intoxication may double a driver's risk of a car crash. Moreover, those who smoke heavily develop lung damage that may prove irreversible.

There is also the issue of impairment in learning, especially in young smokers consuming it extensively as teens. When smoking in young adolescence, this results in impaired brain development, along with poorer performance in school.

As demonstrated by investigators in the *Journal of Neuroscience* marijuana causes actual structural changes in the brain of young adults, aged 18 through 25. The two areas which suffered these defects are the nucleus accumbens and the amygdala. This was seen in those using the drug at least once per week.

It is adolescents who suffer the worst. Users are more likely to do poorly in school and even drop out versus non-users. In a New Zealand study it was found that regular teen users suffered a drop in IQ of some eight points by the fourth decade. Whether this was a result of smoke inhalation itself or the toxicity of THC was not determined.

Even so, it will be argued by the pro-marijuana group that this book is too harsh on the smoked matter. "It's natural. The body has its own THC receptors for that purpose." This argument is perhaps best dispelled by University College of London's V. Curran, when she said as reported by *Science Daily*, "They (that is the CB1 cannabinoid receptors) are not put there by God, so we can enjoy (smoking) cannabis. They're put there, because we *have our own cannabis in our brains.*"

With the youth, though, it is like all other psychoactive substances. Developing individuals are far more vulnerable to any toxic effects, including long-term damage, than adults. In this regard it should not be taken lightly. Children should never recreationally smoke anything, whether tobacco-based or pot-based, and that includes adolescents.

Even so, who doesn't recall seeing young teens smoking marijuana, often in large groups? It surely wasn't toxic enough to cause long-term brain damage in all such smokers. For many it was merely an experimental drug, just like alcohol. The issue, here, is one of excessive use and also significant long-term use. That is not recommended in the least. Daily smoking, for instance, of any plant matter will result in a degree of toxicity, especially in developing youths. Who could find the regular inhalation of, for instance, wood fire smoke a good thing?

When it is carefully considered, it becomes clear that the smoking of hallucinogenic marijuana should be completely discouraged in young people, in particular. Notes Curran, "Kids are growing up on a much more toxic form of marijuana than they would have done years ago." Today's plants are very high in THC and low in...cannabidiol, or CBD," which counteracts its effects. According to a marijuana potency study at the University of Mississippi THC levels in marijuana have increased from 3.4 percent in 1993 to 8.8 percent in 2008. Surely, the nearly 9% matter would prove highly addictive for teenage smokers.

Even so, is there a positive side to smoking for the world's youth? It's not the world's youth, really, since, curiously, the majority of recreational smoking occurs in America and Europe as well as other Westernized regions. How common, for instance, is its use in the young people of Africa, the Middle East, Mexico, and Central America? In fact, the consumption or smoking of recreational marijuana there is rare.

So, are there special needs of such Westernized youth which makes pot smoking a positive thing? Surely, for young people smoking any substance habitually cannot be productive. Pot smoking has more derogatory consequences than positive ones, so it should be at all costs avoided. It creates an apathetic, if not dysfunctional, nature. In particular, young people should not utilize habit-forming, psychoactive substances, whether pot, alcohol, illicit drugs, or other.

Most youths experiment with pot and then, ultimately, abandon it. In such individuals there are usually no long-term negative consequences. In this respect even in the scientific community no one can say with confidence that such moderate or short-term marijuana use is toxic. One reason is the means to determine such toxicity. It is unethical to randomly assign a study where participants use such a banned drug for months, merely so scientists can comprehend the effects. So, there are, essentially, no long-phase studies in human volunteers. Moreover, once again, since it is rather than a refined drug an actual plant substance or herb it is less aggressive, and less destructive, than the obviously and more heavily refined toxins, alcohol, cocaine, codeine, and heroin. With the latter the toxicity is readily defined and is proven through scientific studies.

One of the strongest links found thus far comes from studies of young people. The teenage brain is still growing and refining its neural connections — a process that's regulated in part by the brain's natural endocannabinoid system. Marijuana use when the brain is vulnerable may interfere with its normal development. Notes one investigator, K. L. Franson: "The developing brain is at risk." It could not get more clear and basic than this.

So, then, if these are the issues, what is the 'good' of smoking recreational, hallucinogenic pot? It is a mood-altering substance and, thus, may temporarily aid in the relief of stress, causing a mellowing out sensation. This, though, is a false front. It doesn't allow the smoker to face the reality of the situation and deal with it in a rational fashion. Therefore, this isn't ultimately a 'good' consequence. Then, there is the issue of pharmacological effects: reduction in pain and muscle spasms. This is a positive result, because it amounts to a kind of sedation or analgesic action: a drug-like action for people in chronic pain, just like codeine or other opiates. Yet, all such positive actions can be achieved through the intake of the industrial species of hemp without the slightest risk for addiction or side effects. Thus, with few exceptions there is no purpose for psychoactively bred marijuana.

Even so, the purpose, here, is not to be "anti-marijuana." Rather, it is merely to give a realistic, balanced view. It is also to warn about the potential negative consequences from long-term use of the substance. People should know the facts at-hand and not be bamboozled by misinformation.

For adults the toxicity is not as clear, at least in the scientific model. Most of the negative effects of marijuana—poorer attention, working memory and mental nimbleness—were absent in adults who quit or had not used the drug for a month, investigators have discovered. However, in some studies it has been determined that a person's ability to plan and make complicated decisions are still impaired a month out, indicating there could be long-term damage.

In real life, though, it is more obvious, as demonstrated by the following case history:

CASE HISTORY: Mr. T., a famous British musician, had smoked pot regularly for some 40 years. As a result, he was in a state of poor health. He suffered lung damage and his memory was disrupted as was his overall energetics. Apathy had set in; his work performance suffered.

There was a bluish tone to his nail beds due to oxygen deprivation. It was obvious that he had been negatively affected; the musician was fully oxygen-deprived and largely dysfunctional: and his friends well knew it. He was flatly told that he must quit the habit, while supplements were supplied to help him do so. Yet, he was so severely addicted that he refused to change and, thus, he continued with the habit and saw little to no improvement in his condition.

Here is another issue. High THC marijuana has been combined, notably in various shops in Colorado and California, with chocolate and cane sugar. That makes three stimulants or, rather, drug agents together. This is never a good idea. In Colorado, where laws regarding marijuana, have been loosened, a number of children under 12 have been admitted to ER rooms for acute marijuana toxicity. This is largely from the overconsumption of cookies and chocolates infused with the substance. In this regard many marijuana shops are essentially 'sweet shops,' selling items far more addictive than candy itself.

Yet, let us be realistic. Despite any issues of reactions and danger serious toxicity is, admittedly, less common than with the 'legal,' commonly consumed drugs, alcohol and tobacco. To skew this fact, though, there are marijuana apologists, who write all sorts of nonsense such as this report, as follows:

At San Francisco General Hospital 5000 acute drug intoxications were treated in 1967. Despite the high incidence of marijuana use in San Francisco, no "marijuana psychoses" were seen. In fifteen months of operation the Haight-Ashbury Clinic has seen approximately 30,000 patient-visits for a variety of medical and psychiatric problems. Our research indicated that at least 95% of the patients had used marijuana...no case of primary marijuana psychosis was seen.

Perhaps there is some truth to it. Yet, it should be kept in mind that this was recorded in the 1960s and 1970s. Today's marijuana is significantly more toxic, partly because of the way it is bred and also because of the chemicals that are used in its production.

Then, what in marijuana can make a person sick? It's not just the THC. It must be kept in mind that it is grown haphazardly under suspect conditions. Much of it is grown indoors, largely because it is raised clandestinely. With rare exceptions this is true even of so-called medical marijuana. As stated in *Mother Jones* magazine it can be tainted by mold and can also contain the shedding from animals, particularly from guard dogs, like pit bulls. Whether grown indoors or outdoors it may be corrupted with residues of synthetic fertilizers and also, possibly, herbicide residues. It's the nature of the cannabis plant. It readily catches or traps such materials, particularly the sticky, gooey resin.

There is another key issue. Some of it is fertilized with dung and in some cases even composted human feces. Residues of such matter have been measured in particular on indoor grown marijuana. With street-bought pot there are no controls. Then, people are going to smoke such matter? The danger to human health is obvious.

As described in *Annals of Allergy, Asthma, & Immunology*, 2015, there is another issue associated with the man-made type. This is allergy to the plant's pollen and also to its smoke. Allergic reactions can be manifested by runny nose, itching and swelling about the eyes, coughing, sneezing, and even hives.

Yet, these are also the symptoms of mold intolerance. Mold readily grows on any green that is improperly dried and, in fact, indoor-raised pot is particularly vulnerable. To smoke such moldy pot would prove disastrous to health.

Even so, it is possible to be reactive to hemp itself, even if organic even the industrial kind. This is true of virtually any plant; people can have allergic propensities. In one case a person who consumed seafood encrusted with hemp seed experienced anaphylactic shock, which can prove fatal. This was likely a result of a combined reaction to the seafood plus the hemp.

Like any pollenating plant allergy is a real concern. In one study, also published in the Annals, up to 45% of those living in hemp-growing areas proved reactive to the pollen. Allergic propensity to the plant is greatly reduced through the powers of wild oregano extract, one of the most potent antihistamines and anti-allergy substances known. In fact, oil of wild oregano is a decided cure against hives as well as anaphylactic shock. This is why it is so ideal to combine hemp extract with the wild oregano.

Is marijuana really criminal?

What is the realistic picture with marijuana? To some degree it is incredible that it is under such draconian laws. Even more incredible is the degree of punishments meted out to the sellers and users. For instance, as far as a crime-producing substance it cannot compare to alcohol, the latter being associated with murder and rape. Furthermore, of the commonly available or used drugs and intoxicants it is the least toxic. Consider the list as published by Lachenmeier and Rehm in *Scientific Reports* from most toxic to least noxious:

- alcohol, including wine
- heroin

- cocaine
- nicotine
- MDMA
- methamphetamine
- methadone
- amphetamine
- diazepam
- THC

Many of these are hard-core drugs. Why is THC so low? This primarily is in respect to the potential for a deadly overdose. Regarding alcohol, which is highest, it is well known that a person can die suddenly, even overnight, from massive intake of the substance. The same is true of heroin.

Yet, it is not a free pass for the drug. Once again, young people are the most vulnerable group. For instance, illicit marijuana use may cause sudden death in youths, in this case 20-some-year olds. According to a study published in *Forensic Science International* two young men in Germany died after taking marijuana. In some cases middle-aged men prove vulnerable. A French study by E. Jouanjus is a case in point. Says Jouanjus, in previous research his group "identified several remarkable cases of cardiovascular complications...in young marijuana users." The finding, he notes, "was unexpected" and, thus, deserved further analysis.

Researchers analyzed serious cardiovascular events or complications following the smoking of the drug, as reported in France's addiction recording network. They identified 35 cases of complications related to the heart, brain, and extremities.

Their findings are as follows:

- the average age of the users was approximately 35 years
- of all nearly 2000 complications some 2% were cardiovascular, a significant number
- of this number of 40 people there were 20 heart attacks, which is highly disconcerting
- there were three reactions related to the brain's arteries
- the rest were related to impaired blood flow in the extremities
- some nine patients died or 25%

The conclusion of the investigators is compelling, which is that cardiovascular reactions and related deaths from pot smoking are under-reported. This is a crucial issue. In France alone there are nearly a million and a half regular users. How many people younger ones in particular with sudden cardiovascular complications are misdiagnosed and are actually marijuana intoxicated?

Once again, here is the issue. People have been *led to believe* that marijuana is non-toxic to the cardiovascular system. There are numerous claims on the Internet that there is no way cannabis can harm the heart or for that matter the brain or arterial system. How can this be? The smoking of any substance causes harm to the cardiovascular system, as well as the brain, if for no other reason than the noxious gases that are produced. According to Jouanjus in summary:

> There is now compelling evidence on the growing risk of marijuana-associated adverse cardiovascular effects, especially in young people. It is therefore important that doctors, including cardiologists, be aware of this and consider marijuana use as one of the potential causes of cardiovascular disorders.

Even so, there are hundreds of other studies, and numerous proclamations, that by no means does the substance play any role in heart disease. Yet, how does this make sense? To smoke a vegetation item and to inhale that smoke is to increase the content of carbon monoxide, as well as carbon dioxide, in the blood, both of which are noxious to the heart. Repeatedly, it has been found that it has a toxicity, raising heart rate as high as double. Though rarely, this could trigger sufficient stress on the heart to cause either a heart attack or cardiac arrhythmia, both of which could be fatal.

Yet, who wants to take such a risk? Says W. Abraham, cardiologist, Ohio State University's Wexner Medical Center it is "not uncommon for us to see marijuana smokers or who ingest marijuana in other forms, in edible forms, come to the ER with anxiety or agitation associated with heart racing."

It also raises blood pressure, an effect seen often directly after its use. Other herbs have this capacity, for instance, thyme and oregano. Yet, the combination of a racing heart plus an increase in blood pressure may be too much for those with weak hearts or other vulnerabilities.

Consider a man who was in his mid-40s, smoking marijuana every night. According to close friends he wasn't a drinker and didn't use any other drugs. Though he was in overall good health one night while smoking pot he had a heart attack and died. Did pot cause it? Circumstantial evidence would indicate that this is the case.

Regardless, it's simply too much stress on the system to cause a sudden, rapid rise in heart rate to this degree. One user, an 18 year-old, reported after heavy smoking that his heart rate rose as high as 150 beats per minute. Obviously, the heart is stressed in the attempt to purge the smoke-induced chemicals from the body.

Make no mistake about it synthetic pot is far more poisonous to the heart than the herbal type, as demonstrated by a study published in 2011 in *Pediatrics*. Here, it was found that three youths, 16 year-olds, suffered heart attacks shortly after smoking the substance known as K2 or spice. Of note, such complexes consist of a combination of herbs and spices laced with synthetically produced cannabinoids.

All three teenagers were seen at Dallas' University of Texas Southwestern Medical Center, where the MIs were confirmed. While the youths had smoked marijuana off and on that week, the heart attacks occurred just after their use of K2. Two tested positive for THC, while negative for all other drugs, including alcohol. No one had determined for certain what it was in this street drug which caused the heart attacks. Even so, such potentially fatal attacks are ultra-rare in this age group. How rare it is for such youths to have myocardial infarctions from any other cause.

K2 or Spice is also known as "incense" or "potpourri," while it is simultaneously listed as "not intended for human use." Within these are found synthetic psychoactive compounds of considerable toxicity. There can be no doubt that they are killer agents. Therefore, officially, synthetic cannabinoid-laced drugs are clearly a cause of both strokes and heart attacks in otherwise healthy adults. They are also hardcore hallucinogens.

It is possible that it is more than merely the smoke or THC that can lead to heart damage. Apparently, in some people the marijuana drugs can so overload the heart as to cause it to stop beating. As published in *Forensic Science International* in a case study a person with a congenitally weak heart was found to suffer a potentially fatal consequence of pot smoking. This is known as cardiac asystole or complete stoppage of the heart muscle from pumping. This is highly serious, because it means that for that time period there is no perfusion of blood to the heart through the coronary arteries. The case, a 21 year-old student, was provided with a Holter monitor where it was found that he had multiple pauses in heart pumping, some lasting as long as 6 seconds. All such pauses were related to the inhalation of the drug. After halting the marijuana the cardiac asystole ceased.

Even so, it is said by the proponents, "Wait a minute, weed", as it is called in slang, "is a natural thing. It's an herb. There's no way it could harm you. As soon as you quit it all goes away. It's all lies." Sure it is, and the nature of human physiology is a lie, too. The fact is the regular smoking of any substance, even the finest, healthiest herb, is never a good idea. To burn up all the healthy components of a substance into smoke and then inhale it and to do so daily or weekly, how can this be healthy? How can it be safe if done on a daily or weekly basis?

Moreover, contrary to any such claim pot is not entirely natural. The type which is smoked has been corrupted. It is bred to be hallucinogenic. Furthermore, unless the person grows it himself, no one knowns what they are getting. Is such a one also smoking and inhaling residues of artificial fertilizers, fungicides, and herbicides? Is dog hair and dander being volatilized and inhaled? What about mold? Are mycotoxins being inhaled and/or ingested with every dose of the substance? The facts are undeniable. As in the regular use of alcohol there are no benefits in the routine, recreational smoking of pot. Long term, the only possible consequence is human harm.

Chapter Six

Cannabinoids to the Rescue

For countless centuries humankind has relied on hemp for its medicinal properties. There was no cabal at that time to fight against it or to restrict its use. Today, there are powerful vested interests which seek to prevent the popularization of medicinal hemp. This is senseless. No other medicinal herb is placed under such scrutiny or pressure.

It is not that modern medicine is against hemp/cannabis as a therapeutic agent: far from it. Synthetic versions of the active ingredients are available as prescription drugs, primarily for the treatment of the side effects of chemotherapy. This means that the medical hierarchy is pro-hemp, even pro-cannabis. This is true if it is this hierarchy which directly profits from the substance. The objective is to own the monopoly on hemp active ingredients, either as refined extracts or synthetic similars. Yet, in therapeutic powers such synthetic or refined versions are relatively impotent compared to the natural, whole—and crude—unprocessed form. Moreover, these synthetic versions are not nearly as diverse, since the whole food form has vastly more powers against a wide range of diseases.

It is the crudeness, the unprocessed whole, that is the secret to the ultimate power of this plant. The same is true of other cannabinoid-rich complexes such as wild rosemary, hops, black pepper, and oregano. For instance, no one seeks to isolate only one or two ingredients of these plants at the expense of all others. It is also the rawness that is crucial. Untarnished hemp cannabinoids are by far the most active, that is compared to the heat-treated and/or solvent-extracted ones. Essentially, these raw forms are flexible or maleable, making them ideal for attaching to human cell membranes. When they are heated, they become altered, kinked and, therefore, are not so vigorous in their ability to attach, that is to the various cannabinoid receptor sites. For optimal therapeutic results hemp extract should always be consumed raw, and this is true also of hemp seed oil, which is considerably damaged through heating.

This is a crucial issue. Hemp is an oily plant, and those oils in raw form are corruption-free. As soon as excesses of heat are applied make no mistake about it the oil molecules will be altered. The molecules are rendered from their natural, maleable, and flexible state to stiff molecules which cannot readily act biochemically, at least not optimally so. This relates to the nature of both these molecules and the brain itself, in fact, that key brain component, the blood-brain barrier. It is well established that the active components of hemp, the cannabinoids, readily pass through that virtually impermeable barrier. This is because cannabinoids are phenolic compounds, specifically, phenolic terpenes, and such compounds efficiently pass into fatty tissue. They are highly flexible and can, essentially, worm their way through the barrier. Even so, it is in the raw state that they are in their ultimate flexible state. The application of any amount of heat alters this, and surely the heat necessary to smoke marijuana does so severely. Additionally, alcohol corrupts the phenolic terpene molecules, and, thus, alcohol-based tinctures are not advised.

This does not mean that heated marijuana or hemp or even the solvent-extracted types is useless. It just means that the fully raw type is optimally active and, thus, most thoroughly effective. This is also the safest type to use and the most well tolerated with essentially zero side effects.

Raw, crude, unprocessed hemp—as the whole CO_2-extracted hemp complex—is one of the most sophisticated, invaluable natural medicines known, especially for the nervous system and brain. Nothing can induce cell regeneration in brain tissue to a greater degree than this complex. Then, when it is combined with crude, raw, wild oregano CO_2 extract, the power and efficacy for disorders of the brain, including actual brain damage, is unsurpassed.

With time, the brain will degenerate. Who in this world would seek to have an intact body, while the brain is absolutely dysfunctional? It would be the most wretched way to live conceivable. Who can fathom it? There is a person who is able to walk, eat, drink, and sleep yet who cannot function mentally to any degree and cannot even remember his own name or the names of his loved ones. This is a sign of endocannabinoid deficiency and also a lack of the ingestion of sufficient amounts of dietary cannabinoids. In the wild animals consume sufficient amounts. No wonder they are free of neurodegenerative diseases.

Yet, this is only part of the issue. Cannabinoids are crucial not only for the central nervous system but also for the endocrine, cardiovascular, and immunological systems. Then, clearly, all people would benefit from daily or routine intake. It is thus necessary to determine the degree of need and deficiency. This can be achieved through an analysis of symptoms and dietary habits. Take the following cannabinoid deficiency self-test to see where you stand:

Cannabinoid deficiency self-test

Which of these applies to you (each test worth one point unless stated otherwise)?

- sleeplessness or insomnia (add 2 points)
- hard time falling asleep, that is lay in bed awake
- anxiety (add 2 points)
- obsessive-compulsive syndrome
- schizophrenia
- seizures or seizure syndrome
- suffering from epilepsy for many years
- taking anti-seizure medications
- taking mood-controlling medications such as SSRIs (add 2 points)
- taking mood-altering medications such as SSRIs for over five years (add 2 points)
- fits of rage and/or anger
- autism/Tourette's/ADHD (add 2 points)
- get too emotional
- lack balance in life
- rarely consume or use spices (add 2 points)
- rarely eat dark leafy greens

- eat mostly meat and potatoes
- do not use CO_2-extracted hemp or whole food hemp oil (add 2 points)
- agitation
- depression
- suicidal thoughts
- drug addiction (add 2 points)
- alcohol addiction (add 2 points)
- suffer from inflammatory condition such as fibromyalgia or arthritis
- autism
- tremors
- hormonal imbalances
- multiple sclerosis
- Lou Gehrig's disease (ALS)
- Parkinson's disease
- chronic pain syndrome
- memory loss
- dementia-like syndrome
- diagnosis of Alzheimer's disease
- family history of dementia
- spinal stiffness and/or inflammation
- weakened immune system
- suffer from glaucoma
- having a hard time coming up with words
- tendency to develop cancer
- significant family history of cancer development
- currently have cancer
- readily develop skin cancer and/or precancerous lesions
- use a cell phone or Wi-Fi on a regular basis
- heavy user of computers and lap-tops and/or video games, including extensive use at night

- under extreme mental/psychological stress (add 2 points)

Your score _____

1 to 4: Possible cannabinoid deficiency

It is possible that you are well compensated for any deficiency. Or, perhaps, you are getting sufficient cannabinoids in the diet, or your body is able to make sufficient amounts. Even so, for optimal health it is advisable to increase the consumption of dark leafy greens, particularly parsley, and also to consume greater quantities of cannabinoid-rich spices. In addition, take a mixture of raw, organic CO_2-extracted hemp plus CO_2-extracted wild oregano, five drops daily.

5 to 8: Mild to moderate cannabinoid deficiency

You are likely not getting sufficient cannabinoids in the diet, and/or your body is unable to make sufficient amounts. For optimal health increase the consumption of dark leafy greens, especially parsley, and also consume greater quantities of cannabinoid-rich spices, including black pepper, rosemary, oregano, basil, hops, cloves, and sage. In addition, take a mixture of raw, organic CO_2-extracted hemp plus CO_2-extracted wild oregano, five to 10 drops daily.

9 to 13: Severe cannabinoid deficiency

You are not consuming enough cannabinoids in the diet, and your body is insufficient in internal production. There is potentially great danger to the body in the event of uncorrected deficiency. To correct this greatly increase the consumption of dark green leafy vegetables, emphasizing parsley, and also various cannabinoid-rich spices, including black pepper, rosemary, oregano, basil, hops, cloves, and sage. Increase the consumption of carrots and carrot juice. Take crude wild oregano capsules with *Rhus coriaria*, two capsules twice daily. Also, take a wild, raw oregano/hemp CO_2-extracted complex, 10 or more drops twice daily. Add a spice-oil fortified hempseed oil supplement to the diet, one T. daily.

14 to 18: Extreme cannabinoid deficiency

Your body is severely deficient in cannabinoids from a lack of sufficient intake and also from defective internal synthesis. Thus, there is potentially great danger here to the body in the event of an uncorrected deficiency. Surely, the body is lacking in the production of its own cannabinoids in sufficient amounts to create the necessary neurological signaling for optimal health. Thus, in addition to increased dietary intake it is necessary to boost the synthesis of endocannabinoids. Greatly increase the consumption of dark green leafy vegetables, particularly parsley, and also various cannabinoid-rich spices, including wild oregano, wild rosemary, wild sage, black pepper, cloves, hops, and basil. Increase the consumption of carrots and carrot juice. Take crude wild oregano capsules with *Rhus coriaria*, three capsules twice daily. Also, take a wild, raw oregano/hemp CO_2-extracted complex, 10 or more drops twice daily. Add a spice-oil fortified hempseed oil supplement to the diet, one T. daily. Also, increase the consumption of grass-fed meat foods, as these are dense sources of arachidonic acid, the precursor to the endocannabinoids.

19 to 24 points: profoundly extreme cannabinoid deficiency

Your body is extremely deficient in cannabinoids from a lack of sufficient intake and also from defective internal synthesis.

Thus, there is potential great danger here to the body in the event of an uncorrected deficiency. Surely, the body is lacking in the production of its own cannabinoids in sufficient amounts to create the necessary neurological signaling for optimal health. Thus, in addition to increased dietary intake it is necessary to boost the synthesis of endocannabinoids. Greatly increase the consumption of dark green leafy vegetables, particularly parsley, and also various cannabinoid-rich spices, including black pepper, basil, wild rosemary, wild sage, cinnamon, cloves, hops, and wild oregano. Increase the consumption of carrots and carrot juice. Take crude wild oregano capsules with *Rhus coriaria*, three capsules twice daily. Also, take a wild, raw oregano/hemp CO_2-extracted complex, 20 or more drops twice daily. Add a spice-oil fortified hempseed oil supplement to the diet, two T. daily. Also, increase the consumption of grass-fed meat foods, as these are dense sources of arachidonic acid, the precursor to the endocannabinoids.

25 and above: Extraordinarily, profoundly extreme cannabinoid deficiency

Your body is deficient to the maximum extreme in cannabinoids from a lack of sufficient intake and also from defective internal synthesis. Thus, there is potentially great danger here to the body in the event of an uncorrected deficiency. Surely, the body is lacking in the production of its own cannabinoids in sufficient amounts to create the necessary neurological signaling for optimal health. Thus, in addition to increased dietary intake it is necessary to boost the synthesis of endocannabinoids. Greatly increase the consumption of dark green leafy vegetables, particularly parsley, and also various cannabinoid-rich spices, including black pepper, basil, wild rosemary, wild sage, hops, cloves, cinnamon, and wild oregano. Increase the consumption of carrots and carrot juice. Take crude wild oregano capsules with *Rhus coriaria*, three capsules twice daily. Also, take a wild, raw oregano/hemp CO_2-extracted complex, 25 or more drops twice daily. Add a spice-oil fortified hempseed oil supplement to the diet, two T. daily. Also, increase the consumption of grass-fed meat foods, as these are dense sources of arachidonic acid, the precursor to the endocannabinoids.

Clearly, then, cannabinoid deficiency is far more common than people realize. It must be in many respects regarded as a deficiency syndrome. At a minimum the deficiency increases the person's vulnerability for the development of serious disease, especially cancer, neurological disorders, disorders of inflammation and heart disease. It also increases the risk for long-term dependancy upon drugs, whether prescription or illicit.

Without the native signalling system within the body the ability of the body systems to be in balance is lost. At all costs that signalling must be restored. This is by boosting the synthesis of naturally occurring cannabinoids and also consuming dietary similars. It is also through activity, since exercise, particularly under sunlight and in fresh air, greatly bolsters internal cannabinoid synthesis.

The modern lifestyle creates major imbalances in the endocannabinoid system. There is stress in general, and there is also electromagnetic stress, that is the toxicity from cell phones, electromagnetic waves, and Wi-fi. In addition, computers have a noxious effect on users; those who use them constantly will deepen the degree of the deficiency. All such electronically exposed individuals would benefit vastly by the use of cannabinoid-rich supplements.

Chapter Seven

The CBD Revolution?

There is a type of marijuana free of any psychoactive properties, that is devoid of the propensity for addiction. This is the species known as industrial hemp, the one used for the making of rope, paper, and other matter. With this type of marijuana there is no risk of addiction. From it is made even food-like products: hempseed protein and hempseed oil. Additionally, there are special kinds of plant concentrates, medicinal complexes, achieved through extraction. One such extraction is commonly known as CBD. This is merely an abbreviation for cannabidiol. It is also known as CBD oil. It is CBD oil which is of major interest in the scientific community for its therapeutic actions in a wide range of diseases, including cancer.

Yet, this itself is an anomaly. CBD implies cannabidiol or shall it be said cannabidiol concentrate. This substance is a terpene, merely one of dozens upon dozens of active ingredients found in the hemp extract complex.

People have been led to believe that CBD is the issue. It is not. The true therapeutic potential is not in the form of an isolate or concentrate but, rather, within the whole, unprocessed complex.

A volatile complex, cannabis is a curious plant. Heat largely corrupts it. Thus, any therapeutic extract for long-term use must be in the raw state.

People have apparently been confused. They see the marketing hype and read the relevant research. They see the significant amount of studies regarding cannabidiol, those studies being marked with the term "CBD" or "CBD oil." Much of this has been done by the pharmaceutical industry to give support to patented drugs. These drugs are based on CBD in the form of cannabidiol.

Cannabidiol is a relatively simple molecule to synthesize, being a basic terpene with phenolic rings. It is as mentioned previously one of some 66 different cannabinoids found in hemp extract. In a high quality industrial hemp extract it might amount to from 10% to 18% of the volume of the whole food fraction. It is worthy to note that nature places Beta-caryophyllene as the primary component of yet another fraction, the aromatic terpene one, making it 50% of the total. The remainder of this fraction consists of novel terpene molecules such as limonene, pinene, and linalool. These latter terpenes are highly volatile and readily driven off by heat.

Then, this is about not merely CBD oil but, rather, in fact, crude hemp leaf/stalk oil, where CBD is merely one of countless other components. This makes the whole, raw, unprocessed complex nothing other than an herbal concentrate. In other words, it is more well described as a plant extract rather than a drug. The intake of a wild oregano oil-fortified raw, whole hemp extract changes the paradigm entirely. This is from one of a highly scrutinized concentrate, CBD oil, that seemingly competes with the drug cartel to be a mere food, a whole plant substance that is absolutely harmless and can only cause benefit. That benefit is an overall improvement in health as well as the treatment and prevention of chronic, degenerative disease.

Moreover, in herbal medicine this is the key, that is a combination of safety and efficacy. With miscellaneous CBD oil supplements no such firm guarantee can be given. It is not that CBD oil doesn't have a value; it certainly does. Yet, when dealing with a dietary supplement, it is crucial to have a high standard for human use. People expect such supplements to at a minimum be harmless and at a maximum to aid them in their quest for optimal health: without side effects. The crude extract achieves this. Is the same true of CBD?

In fact, despite a high profile of safety, overall, there are reports of issues with this form. This is particularly true if the plant has been bred for high cannabidiol levels. For human use a higher density of this substance at the expense of all others is far from ideal, some cultivars having as high as 40% content.

In modern research the history of the molecule is relatively new. First isolated from cannabis in 1940 it took some 20 years to identify its structure, after which it was extensively researched. By 2000 cannabidiol had been defined as a potential therapeutic agent in the treatment of neurosis, particlarly anxiety and psychosis, as well as for epilepsy. It was also being studied as a potential sedative or relaxant. Now, it is being studied for its additional properties such as anti-tumor actions and its capacity to fight inflammation. As demonstrated by investigators publishing in *Current Drug Safety* it was also found to be effective in protecting brain tissue and nerve cells in general from oxidative damage. This led to further research showing potential benefits for dementia, diabetes, and psychiatric disorders.

Even so, in terms of organ systems CBD is a 'safe' cannabinoid devoid of any known serious toxicity. In fact, in some individuals it acts as an anti-toxin, for instance, helping reverse the anxiety or panic attacks caused by marijuana smoking.

It is a strong substance, which acts directly on certain brain centers involved in anxiety, notably the limbic and paralimbic centers. In human volunteers it was found to do the astonishing, which was to reduce anxiety associated with public speaking. This led the researchers publishing in *Neuropsychopharmacology* to deem it an effective therapy for the anxiety which occurs in relation to social events, the so-called SAD or Social Anxiety Disorder. This was achieved with a single dose, which, incredibly, on its own reduced public-speaking-related phobias. Yet, virtually all the healthy cannabinoids have this effect, though cannabidiol may be more potent in this regard.

In another study the substance was found to exert a positive action on cancer, in this case cancelling the powers of a cancer-promoting gene. Cannabidiol has the ability to shut down the gene, known as ID-1. This causes cancer cells to lose their ability to spread or metastasize. High levels of ID-1 have been found in leukemia patients and also within pancreatic, ovarian, brain, colon, rectal, and lung tissues.

Yet, then, how credible is this drug company-sponsored research? It does have a degree of substance. Yet, is it that simplistic, that is merely finding a single active ingredient and researching it, then putting it on the market as a synthetic analogue? Far more sophisticated is to use the whole, crude, raw extract, which includes naturally occurring amounts of CBD but which also contains all other cannabinoids known. This is the future of cannabis therapy. There is no additional value of merely isolating cannabidiol alone, and then of refined or extracted cannabidiol is highest of all at over $10,000 per kilo. This would place CBD therapy out of reach for many people.

Are high-CBD oils ideal?

It makes no sense to ultra-refine any herb. There is no added benefit in this. In fact, such ultra-refinement can lead to untoward effects, including highly distressing side effects. This is because of man-made manipulation. For instance, there is nothing inherently wrong with cannabidiol. Yet, if it is concentrated, it can, when consumed, be overwhelming in its actions. Unfortunately, in the CBD oil trade such ultra-refinement is commonly used. This is in order to concentrate cannabidiol fractions, which are much sought after and command significantly high prices.

Cannabidiol is a potent natural medicine. However, its greatest value is when it is in combination with its synergistic, balancing compounds, that is all the other 450-plus hemp plant substances. Reactions to pure CBD or powerful concentrates can occur. This is the result of artificially manipulating the CBD oil, not any inherent toxicity of cannabidiol. Such reactions include lethargy, heaviness of the limbs, listlessness, nausea, cold body temperature, and puffiness. There may be what is called a "bad drug feeling or hangover."

In addition, a number of serious side effects have been reported, related to certain brands, these effects mostly relating to the intestinal system. Consider the so-called pure CBD oil and/or high cannabidiol CBD oil. Without mentioning brands a number of individuals, children and adults, have suffered significant reactions, often digestive in nature, from such oils. Some have been hospitalized as a result of such reactions. These reactions include nausea, vomiting, cramps, pain in the gut, vomiting, and diarrhea. By no means should a truly natural, whole food hemp oil cause such reactions. It is the concentrates that do so, since by creating such concentrates an aberration occurs.

Such reactions are exceedingly disconcerting, since whole food cannabis extracts do precisely the opposite, which is to balance and stimulate the digestive system, eliminating symptoms rather than causing them. It is possible that such oils are too high in THC, which can cause such digestive distress. Or, they may contain noxious solvents, such as hexane, ethyl alcohol, and isopropyl alcohol, which themselves can lead to digestive reactions, including generalized digestive distress. Some have even been found to contain residues of butane, that is lighter fluid, and ethyl acetate, that is fingernail polish solvent.

It was the Good Samaritan Rick Simpson who first popularized therapeutic marijuana extract, his oil being extracted with solvents. In this regard he freely showed people how they could make it on their own. While this oil has helped a great number of people, still, here solvent extraction is not recommended.

No doubt, cannabidiol is medicinal. Even so, for general use people should not use such a singular substance and/or CBD-fortified oils. To create such oils much refinement is used, including fractional distillation. This leads to a corruption in the molecules. In all cases for regular use only the whole food, raw extract must be consumed for best results. This makes great sense. The full extract has all the components of nature without manipulation, including the highly medicinal terpene molecules: without the slightest degree of alteration.

Chapter Eight

Medical Conditions

There a number of medical conditions which fully respond to cannabinoid therapy. Many of these conditions, such as multiple sclerosis, Parkinson's disease, ALS, epilepsy, and certain types of cancers, are regarded as virtually incurable. In some cases cannabis therapy represents the most potent, effective remedy known. Many such conditions also respond to wild oregano oil therapy, which demonstrates the invaluable nature of a combined approach.

This combined approach is truly novel. Wild oregano acts synergistically with the CO_2 hemp extract. It potentizes it. It also fills the gaps, biochemically, in the hemp profile. As a result, the wild oregano-hemp complex is incomparably more effective as a therapeutic aid than hemp extract alone. Let us evaluate the primary conditions which are positively affected by hemp-wild oregano therapy and which in many instances can be outright reversed. Truly, this treatment is a vast blessing upon humankind and can give great hope, including the hope and potential for a complete cure.

Seizure syndromes

The clinical evidence for the use of cannabinoid-rich herbs, such as cannabis, holy basil, wild sage, wild rosemary, and wild oregano, is vast. Yet, is there any hard scientific research to support this? The largest study to date published by O. Devinsky and his group, was recently (2015) presented at the American Epilepsy Society meeting, with the results being highly significant. Involving some 313 epilepsy victims, all children, the study was initiated in 2014 with patients being monitored over a 90 day period. Of the 261 children who remained in the study virtually all had a response which was astounding: a 50% reduction in seizure or convulsion incidence. Furthermore, some 10% of the participants were seizure-free in that short treatment period.

Now, this was through the use of a specialized cannabinoid drug known as Epidiolex. With this drug there were reports of side effects, though relatively minor. Those side effects included drowsiness, diarrhea, tiredness, and decreased appetite. Surely, the use of the whole, crude unprocessed material, the fully cannabinoid complex, is much more readily tolerated plus far more potent in overall results than a single molecule.

In this regard it is a superior approach to combine like herbal medicines for a more thorough effect, also to treat a wider range of elements. Consider the combination of whole crude CO_2 hemp extract with whole crude CO_2 wild oregano extract. Both are rich sources of cannabinoids; in fact, the combination creates a broader spectrum of such compounds than with cannabis alone. While cannabis contains a wider range of cannabinoids, some 60 in total, wild oregano is a rich source of other key phenolic compounds, such as carvacrol and to a smaller degree thymol, which are devoid in hemp. These phenolic compounds are potent antioxidants, which help activate and preserve the powers of the hemp-based cannabinoids, including caryophyllene. Furthermore, carvacrol and thymol are powerful antiseptics. In many cases epilepsy is caused by infections, including those induced by vaccines. Thus, the combination of wild oregano and hemp extracts covers the range of causative factors far more thoroughly than hemp extract alone.

Consider the investigation published by J. W. Sander, *Infectious Agents and Epilepsy*. Notes Sander a wide range of infectious agents are involved in the causation of seizure syndromes, including the parasites *Toxocara canis* and the beef tapeworm, *Taenia saginata*. The parasitic agent *Echinococcus granulosus* is also correlated. Furthermore, there is evidence the worms *Schistosoma japonicum* and *manoni* are culprits. Regarding protozoa, *Toxoplasma gondii* is associated. All such parasites are capable of invading brain tissue. There, they create cysts, which place pressure on brain centers, leading to seizures.

The pork tapeworm *Taenia solium* is also a major cause of epilepsy. It attacks and consumes brain tissue, where it lays its eggs. The case of the individual with multiple brain cysts associated with seizures is often due to this infestation. Infection of the brain by this parasite with the associated brain cyst or cysts is known as cysticercosis. Untreated, it readily leads to fatality.

Whether beef or pork tapeworm the infection is usually the result of the consumption of uncooked or improperly cooked meat. Another means of contraction is the tainting of cooking or food preparation surfaces with raw meat or its residues.

Pork is particularly dangerous because of the nature of its tapeworms. The cysts of this parasite resist destruction by heat. So, any pork that is not thoroughly cooked, fully well done, can potentially transmit the disease. Regardless, this type of meat is unfit for human consumption and should, in particular, never be consumed by those with seizure syndromes. All the major scriptures have banned this type of meat for sound reason. Pork is a transmitter of a number of diseases, some of which, like trichinosis, are virtually incurable. Then, on what basis should it be consumed?

Fungal organisms, too, may play a role, notably *Candida albicans, Histoplasmosis capsulatum,* and *Cryptococcus neoformans*, as well as the invasive mold mucor. All have been reported in the medical literature as key causes of epileptic seizures. Moreover, all such fungi can in suspectable people readily infect the brain and spinal cord.

Regarding viruses, the number which may be associated is significant. In most cases they operate by stealth with no physical evidence, unless they cause actual inflammation of the brain, for instance, meningitis and/or encephalitis. For instance, the herpes virus may be an unsuspected cause. So can the various vaccine viruses, particularly those injected through the MMR vaccine.

In fact, vaccines or shall it be said septic inoculations are a major cause of seizure syndromes. Can anyone fathom what is happening here? Through the injection of these agents of septic degeneration the normal immune defenses are by-passed. Consider infants and children. No one would ever knowingly subject them to dangerous infectious agents. The fact is people do all they can to protect, for instance, babies and infants from germs. Yet, the world trusts physicians to arbitrarily inject germs unknown into their tissues with direct access to both the bloodstream and the lymph? This makes no sense to any degree.

Here is the key issue. The immune system of the newborn, infant, and/or toddler is weak, underdeveloped. Then, without a strong capacity to respond live pathogens are injected into the body, a number of which readily infect the brain. Contrary to popular belief those germs within the injections truly are alive: with very few exceptions. Upon injection into the body these pathogens seek the means for survival, and that necessitates the invasion of human tissue, including internal organs such as the brain. For instance, one of the main causes of autism, essentially a chronic neurological infection syndrome, is the MMR inoculation which leads to infestation by measles, mumps, and rubella viruses, all of which readily invade and infect brain cells as well as the cells of the spinal cord. The polio immunization, the sugar cube, is infested with highly pathogenic viruses originating from rhesus monkeys, including the so-called Simian Virus 40 or SV40. It is this virus which is known as a neurotropic virus, meaning it has a strong preference and capacity to invade human nervous tissue. SV40 is a primary cause of brain tumors in toddlers and children, and surely in some cases the developing tumorous masses lead to seizures.

Bacteria are a well-established cause of epilepsy. The bacteria known to cause it are largely those which cause meningitis. These bacteria include H. influenza, N. meningitides, and S. pneumoniae, all of which can cause chronic infection of the brain and spinal cord, therefore leading to chronic seizure syndromes.

There can even be infectious abscesses in the brain. These abscesses place pressure on brain cells, leading to seizures. Among the germs which can cause this are a wide range of parasites as well as certain fungi and bacteria. Sinus disorders may also result in abscess formation. The bones covering the sinus cavities are exceedingly thin and can be readily compromised through chronic, long-standing infection. In this case the causative factor is various molds, including red rust mold, green mold, and black mold. The same is true of deep abscesses of the teeth, where the infection may transfer into the brain matter, as the roots of the teeth provide direct access. All such infectious causes are resistant to standard treatments.

Even malaria may lead to infectious seizures. The malarial parasite, *Plasmodium falciparum*, readily infects brain tissue.

Now, as a most revealing finding it was Woodruff who some 30 years ago found a connection between animal parasites and epilepsy. He had determined that the disease was much more common in dog owners than in non-dog owners. The difference in incidence was so significant that he determined dog ownership to be a 'major risk factor.' This is thought to be related to infestation by the dog parasite, *Toxocara canis*. Infestation is more common in low income households and/or societies than in wealthier districts. Even so, virtually anyone can contract the parasite as a result of poor or sloppy hygiene in relationship to dogs and/or their excrement.

In fact, direct contact with dogs can lead to the inoculation. This is particularly true from kissing them or having direct contact of the saliva in the face or hands. One avenue for toxocara for invasion is the eyes. The fact is in poor countries or tribal countries where there is much contact of children with dogs toxocara eye infection is common. Dog saliva also contains viruses which can readily infect the brain stem. By no means should dogs ever be kissed or licked, as this can lead to infection of the brain by seizure-causing pathogens.

Nor should children handle them without following careful hygiene in the aftermath, that is careful hand washing. Nor should children sleep with their dogs. Moreover, regarding dog feces owners must follow fastidious hygiene and be sure to wash the hands thoroughly after handling dog feces.

For epileptic children there is an association with pica or the eating of dirt or soil. This is thought to be due to the ingestion of parasitic cysts, including those of *Toxocara canis*.

Odds are high for the development of epilepsy in those who have evidence of blood infection by the parasite. This is particularly true when serology tests show evidence of current, active infection. In this case the infection must be thoroughly purged from the blood, as well as the rest of the body, for the epilepsy to be cured.

Further studies have been done on this, particularly in so-called cryptogenic epilepsy. The word itself derives from the Greek derivative "kryptos," meaning "hidden." Thus, this type of condition is held as 'cause unknown.' In such cases infection plays a major role. To summarize the types of infectious agents which are associated with the cause of epilepsy and other seizure disorders, as well as virtual epileptic conditions such as tic douloureux and autism, are as follows:

- *Toxocara canis*
- *Toxocara manoni*
- *Toxoplasma gondii*
- *Taenia solium*
- *Taenia saginata*
- *Echinococcus granulosus*

- *Schistosoma japonicum*
- *Schistosoma manoni*
- *Cryptococcus neoformans*
- *Histoplasmosis capsulatum*
- measles virus
- mumps virus
- rubella virus
- herpes virus
- SV40 neurotropic virus
- H. influenza
- N. meningitides
- S. pneumoniae
- *Plasmodium falciparum*

What a vast, if not ominous, list it is. It fully demonstrates the major role of infection in this condition. There are surely numerous other pathogens which are associated. The point is with any approach to this condition an anti-infection purge should be included. Whole food, raw CO_2-extracted hemp oil is surely a key element, but far more powerful is such oil fortified with the potent antiseptic complex, wild, raw CO_2 oregano extract. That is needed to root the parasites out of the brain and the rest of the body. Yet, regardless of the cause in all cases of epilepsy the combination of raw extract of wild oregano and hemp should be applied, since to a degree seizures represent a defect in the endocannabinoid system.

Yet, there are a number of other chronic neurological conditions where infection may play the most predominant role. These neurological conditions which respond to hemp-wild oregano therapy include depression, anxiety, obsessive-compulsive syndrome, psychosis, schizophrenia, dementia,

Parkinson's disease, multiple sclerosis, ALS, Alzheimer's disease, autism, trigeminal neuralgia, brain cancer, and tic douloureux. Few if any people would consider these infectious conditions, and physicians surely rarely if ever do so. All such conditions will likely respond to the hemp-oregano oil combination.

Whether for such neurological conditions or chronic pain disorders, long term, smoking cannabis is not the answer for neurological pain and inflammation. That's because, long term, smoking itself is pro-inflammatory. Furthermore, THC and its metabolites can cause damage to brain cells. For this reason it should not be consumed except, perhaps, as a short-term agent. In contrast, the combination of organic CO_2 hemp from industrial species, along with wild, raw oregano oil extract, is absolutely safe for daily consumption. Even so, it is powerful enough that in some instances occasional consumption, like two or three times per week, is sufficient.

No doubt, oil of wild oregano is the most potent natural germ killer known. It is particularly effective against viruses, bacteria, molds, and yeasts. Regarding parasites, as published in the scientific literature its main action is against protozoans: amebas, blastocystis, cryptosporidium, the malarial parasite, and giardia. It is also an ideal agent for brain infections of any type, as many of its components penetrate the blood-brain barrier.

Even so, for major infestations and for infections by larger parasites, such a tape worms and flukes, often it is necessary to add other antiparasitic complexes. The total body purging agent is one such complex. Consisting of wild, raw greens extracts, including the highly cleansing wild, raw burdock, nettles, and dandelion extracts, it is fortified with the powers of antiparasitic black seed oil, bay leaf oil, sage oil, and fennel oil. It also contains wild, raw dandelion root, which is a potent purging agent for the gallbladder, bloodstream, and liver. This complex acts to purge all infectious parasites from the system.

Is there any evidence that wild oregano itself is a remedy for seizures? In fact, historically, it was used precisely for this purpose. It was the ancient Greeks who used it successfully for treating seizure syndromes but also as a cure for other head-related syndromes such as migraines. This was confirmed by Greek investigators, who found in an animal model that, surely, wild oregano is effective at reducing seizures. In the study the investigators, publishing in *Epilepsy Research and Treatment*, found that the essential oil of wild oregano, rich in the active ingredient carvacrol, prevented seizures significantly. So did other essential oils, including oils of mint, peppermint, basil, rosemary, and lavender. Yet, incredibly, in most common medical literature rosemary is banned for use in seizure treatment. One element these oils have in common is that they are all dense sources of the cannabinoid Beta-caryophyllene.

None of the essential oils to any degree caused an increase in seizures. In fact, the oils were so effective that the investigators deemed them "anticonvulsants." One reason for this positive effect is the antiviral powers of the essential oils, wild oregano being the leader in this regard. According to work published in the *Journal of Applied Microbiology*, 2014, oregano oil inactivates viruses rapidly, including the kind capable of infecting human tissue. The virus killing and inhibiting powers were so great that oregano was deemed a virtual sanitizer against viruses and also a natural "antiviral" agent. Other studies, including the work of Siddiqui published in *Medical*

Science Research, prove that oregano oil causes the disintegration of viruses, including those of the herpes family. In work by Ijaz and Ingram it was found that wild oregano oil, using the P73 edible type, caused in rather small doses the near complete destruction of noxious viruses within cells. The cells were infected with trillions of such viruses, and the oregano oil obliterated the intracellular infection, in this case by influenza A, the bird flu virus, and the human coronavirus, all of which can cause potentially fatal encephalitis.

Mold infestation is no minor issue. It is well established that the key poisons from molds, known as mycotoxins, can readily damage the nervous system. This is particularly true of black mold, especially the species known as stachybotrys. The trichothecene mycotoxins produced by this mold are decided neurotoxins. This implies the incredible, which is that they kill nerve cells.

Exposure occurs primarily through breathing the mold spores. The highly poisonous mycotoxins, when inhaled, cause a burning sensation, tightness in the chest, shortness of breath, and burning feelings in the nose, sinuses, and bronchial passages. In some cases the mycotoxins cause bleeding, that is the spitting up of blood. Systemic symptoms of mold poisoning are as follows:

- confusion and brain fog
- disorientation
- dizziness
- memory loss
- impairment of thinking; learning impairment
- poor concentration
- hallucinations

- anxiety and/or depression
- tingling sensations
- trembling
- numbness
- shaking
- seizures

There is significant proof for the role of black mold in seizures as well as other neurological disorders. Consider the investigations at Tufts University. Here, as published in the *Journal of the American Veterinary Association* it was reported that in dogs mold toxins in a single household caused "muscle tremors, trouble walking, and seizures." The existence of the poisons was proven through analysis of the animals' stomach contents, where the noxious agents were identified as penitrem A and roquefortine. Both these mycotoxins are from the green mold penicillium, which had apparently overgrown in the household. It is no easy issue to poison dogs to such a degree, which are highly resilient animals.

In many cases the humans in such tainted homes also develop seizures. In one anecdotal report a woman and her dog suffered seizures after living in a rather cheap apartment building. Ultimately, it was determined that the cause was mold growing in her bathroom and being aerosolized within the attic.

Not every person suffering such a degree of exposure will develop the neurotoxic effects. It is merely another key risk factor that may be responsible for sudden onset seizures in humans and/or animals, particularly in those who have no prior history of the syndrome. Yet, by no means should mycotoxin/mold exposure be treated lightly. No doubt, severe lung disorders, cancer, and heart disease have been associated with prolonged exposure to molds. The lungs are particularly vulnerable, and many "cause unknown" chronic lung disorders are caused primarily by mold. In some cases repetitive and/or massive exposure can prove fatal.

Mold poisons are not only external, that is within the air or embedded within structures, but are also internal. This is the real issue, which is chronic, systemic infection by black or other molds, where the living molds produce mycotoxins within the body. A person can as a result be essentially "autopoisoned" by the internally produced mycotoxins. This demonstrates the importance of wild oil of oregano as a means to reverse this major cause of disorders of the nervous system. There can be nothing more powerful than this oil in reversing mycotoxin poisoning. Research has shown that wild oregano oil is highly destructive to mycotoxins as well as the molds themselves. Within the tissues exposure to the oil causes the destruction of any embedded molds, while also neutralizing their poisons. Additionally, cumin oil is highly effective in neutralizing the toxicity of these poisons. One potent formula, known as OregaRESP, is based on dessicated oils of wild oregano and cumin, along with sage and cinnamon oils. Both sage and cinnamon are potent antifungal agents. This formula would be an ideal adjunct to the hemp oil-oregano-based sublingual drops. Regular intake would cause an improvement in nerve and brain function and, in fact, overall health.

Treatment protocol

To treat this condition take the hemp-wild oregano combination, five or more drops under the tongue or as a single gelcap two or more times daily. For difficult situations take it more frequently, like five or more times daily. Do this until the seizure syndrome stabilizes and then continue a maintenance dose, as needed. For extreme situations use the super-strength form of the hemp-wild oregano complex, five to ten drops as often as needed. For suspicion of infectious causes of seizures or epilepsy take the multiple spice complex, two capsules twice daily, as well as the total body purging agent, one or two ounces daily on an empty stomach or with food/juice. Additionally, avoid the consumption of refined sugar, black tea, coffee, cocoa, and chocolate. Beware of GMO-tainted foods and beverages. These corrupt 'foods' can readily promote seizures. The primary GMOs to avoid are foods tainted with commercial soy and corn as well as beet sugar, canola, and cottonseed.

Insomnia

Cannabinoid- and caryophyllene-rich plants are among the most effective treatments known not only for disorders of the nervous system but also for sleep disorders. This includes intractable insomnia. Sleeplessness or insomnia is a virtual epidemic, afflicting some one-third of all Westerners. The negative effects of this are significant, with significant loss of quality of life and productivity. Here is where whole food cannabinoid sources can prove invaluable. The cannabinoid-rich plants which act as anti-insomnia medications include holy basil, cinnamon, wild oregano, chamomile, hemp, and hops. Regarding hops, this is one of the most sophisticated of all known herbal medicines, Known primarily as a bitters for the flavoring of beer in previous centuries this herb was in antiquity highly prized for its therapeutic properties. It was held in particular significance during medieval times, and this makes sense, since hops are mainly a Northern Hemisphere plant. Here, the herb was fully established as an effective treatment for anxiety disorders, tension, and insomnia. Notes R. Whelan, medical herbalist, it was also dispensed as a remedy for irritated organ systems, specifically "nervous diarrhea, nervous stomach, and nervous bladder."

In Victorian times hops were highly regarded. As noted in Kings Dispensatory, 1898, "Hops are principally used for their sedative..." actions. Is that not a most fascinating issue? With all the drugs available for sleeplessness, as well as hard-core insomnia, the lowly hops are the categorical answer, and it has all been so neglected. The book continues to state that, like drugs, it has a "hypnotic action, producing sleep..." Who, suffering insomnia, would not like to have a bit of non-toxic, herbal hypnotic action? According to these Victorian-era herbalists it was established that hops were effective against agitation and irritation, in fact, all forms of "restlessness" and also as a means for "abating pain."

Said these early researchers the bitter herb was also found to be invaluable for nervous and worry-induced digestive disorders, specifically "dyspepsia" or sour/upset stomach. The hops were thought to act on the nerve centers to ease such stomach upset. It was apparently a mainstay in the treatment of any nervous or otherwise related disorders of the gut, including gastritis and enteritis, the latter indicating inflammatory toxicity of the small intestines. Hemp, too, has many of the same historical uses. This is why a combination of CO_2 extracts of both plants is so ideal.

Even over-agitation, sexually, is responsive to the plant extract. This is in regard to sexual excitability. In fact, it is believed that this was the origin of the use of hops in beer, as the primary beer makers at the time were monks. The addition of hops to beer was mandated in order to minimize sexual desires in the monk population: purportedly to prevent them from "straying" from celibacy. Prior to this it was other bitter herbs, notably dandelion and burdock, that were used in beer flavoring.

The suppression or balancing of sexual desires is thought to be the result of the rich amount of natural estrogen in this plant. By the way, that natural estrogen in modest amounts is non-toxic to humans. In fact, for women hops may prove to be an effective treatment for menopausal syndrome. Moreover, like wild oregano and hemp extract a key active ingredient of hops is the potent cannabinoid Beta-caryophyllene and its related terpenoid molecule, alpha humulene. As well, like hops wild oregano has been used historically as a sleep aid. More recent investigations have determined that it is effective both internally and topically. Wild oregano oil may be used topically as a rub over the chest and lower neck area to effectively induce sleep in a troubled sleeper.

For hops the scientific studies demonstrating efficacy are significant. Consider the work of German investigators Dimpfel and Suter publishing in the *European Journal of Medical Research*. Here, in human subjects it was discovered that extract of hops, in this case combined with valerian extract, induced sleep better than a placebo. The investigators found that the hops/valerian takers fell into a deeper sleep at a much better rate and length of such sleep than the sugar pill takers. Using an EEG to measure the actions through a single administration the herbal therapy proved so effective that the investigators deemed it a "successful" therapy. In other words, the hops acted as a hypnotic agent, just as the early herbalists described. Then, can anyone image its powers when combined with cannabinoid-rich hemp and wild oregano, which are also major hypnotics? It is well known that cannabis, for instance, when smoked, leads to tiredness. This is a result of the direct action of inhaled cannabinoids on neurological centers. This induction of tiredness can prove useful in sleeplessness. It might be said that this is more of a relaxation response than merely making a person exhausted. With high-THC marijuana it is not. Rather, it is a toxicity against the neuromuscular centers which leads to a sensation of heaviness of the body, including the limbs.

In contrast, the other key cannabinoids, the CB2 activating ones, are largely devoid of such reactions. One exception is cannabidiol itself which may overload certain receptor sites, leading to untoward symptoms. This is only an issue with so-called CBD oil. In other words, it is never an issue with the crude, whole food extract. The whole food extract is a balance of all the wide range of cannabinoids, never manipulated, never altered. Rather than creating fatigue or heaviness it does the opposite, increasing natural energy as well as muscular strength.

Even so, CBD-rich hemp leaf and stalk extracts do have novel properties on the brain. In particular, they play a key role in inducing a sense of calm or relaxation. One study found that CBD is more effective in inducing sleep in humans than THC. One explanation for this positive effect of CBD-rich oil relates to the neurotransmitter, serotonin. Cannabinoids cause an increase in this brain cell-modulating chemical. These compounds have even been shown to induce regeneration of brain cells, an essential element in the treatment of intractable insomnia.

Yet another powerful sleep aid is holy basil. Why is it so powerful? Like hops and cannabis the herb is a dense source of cannabinoids, largely in the form of Beta-caryophyllene. It is this substance which most efficiently stimulates the body's cannabinoid receptor sites. Basil also is rich in eugenol and myrcene, which have relaxing powers over the nerves and muscles. These are sedative-like compounds, which are also found in cloves and hops, respectively.

Regardless, basil is a novel herb with much value for health improvement. The herb is well known for its capacity to relieve stress, also for its capacity to boost adrenal function. In this regard it aids in the synthesis of cortisol, a hormone essential for restful sleep. In fact, according to research published by India's Central Drug Research Institute basil helps normalize cortisone production, while also helping to balance/normalize blood sugar. Basil also reduces sensitivity to background noise, essential to healthy sleep. A high noise sensitivity is a sign of adrenal exhaustion. Chewing on a few basil leaves at bedtime can help both in easing adrenal stress and also in sedation.

Its powers in balancing blood sugar are no minor issue. A whole food form of holy basil can be used as a diabetic aid, as it acts on two key organ systems involved in this disease, the adrenal glands and the pancreas. Plus, through its rich content of Beta-caryophyllene it helps calm the nerve centers, which greatly aids in adrenal gland regeneration.

Camomile is another herbal medicine which aids in a calming response. This makes it an ideal sleep aid. Like wild cold-extracted oregano oil and CO_2 hemp extract, it is a healthy source of the nerve modulating agent Beta-caryophyllene. A hot cup of camomile tea is exceedingly relaxing before bedtime. Additionally, the CO_2 extract of this flowering herb is a potent sedative and can be taken in supplemental form as a sleep aid.

In fact, the majority of essential oils act to normalize nerve function, oil of wild oregano being no exception. Oregano oil has additional novel properties. It is a potent analgesic, that is pain relieving agent. It also helps halt and purge inflammation. Furthermore, it possesses muscle relaxing properties. All such functions prove invaluable for the induction of healthy sleep. In fact, a number of the diseases which lead to insomnia are associated with inflammation and/or chronic pain. Obviously, if the pain is relieved, there will be sleep induction.

There have been many instances where this has proven to be the case. The person is suffering with intractable pain with associated inflammation. Nothing can be done to induce sleep, since the nerve centers are agitated as a result of the pathology. Then, when the wild oregano oil is applied topically as well as taken internally, sleeping is induced. Topical application may include rubbing of the oil as an extra virgin olive oil emulsion on the pain area but also doing so on the soles of the feet, the shins, and up-and-down the spine. If it is infection related, there may also be rubbing about the upper rim of the clavicles towards the midline, the purpose being the stimulation of lymph flow. As a result, the person becomes at ease, benefits from a reduction in pain, and falls asleep.

CASE HISTORY: Man with pain-associated insomnia falls asleep after rubbing wild oregano oil on upper chest.

Mr. K. is a 55 year-old man who suffers bouts of chronic pain, along with significant stiffness of the neck and upper back. Attributing it to weakened adrenals he takes nutritional supplements for supporting these hormone glands, which helps, but once the spinal stiffness sets in he finds it impossible to get a good night's rest or even to fall asleep readily at all. He had decided to rub his upper chest with the wild oregano oil and also take the hemp-oregano oil CO_2 extract combination. He also rubbed oregano oil on the soles of his feet. Within 15 minutes he fell asleep and had a sound sleep for the first time in weeks.

Fungal infestation, notably by the yeast *Candida albicans*, is yet another cause of sleeplessness. It is well established that yeast overload leads to nervous irritation, agitation, and in some cases insomnia. The yeast creates toxins, including candida toxin and formaldehyde, which poison the central nervous system. Purging the candida, which both hemp oil extract and, particularly, oil of wild oregano can achieve creates a sensation of calm.

A sleep aid containing a number of these natural, whole herb complexes is now available. Available as sublingual drops this formula is a mixture of CO_2-extracted hemp, along with CO_2 and essential oil extracts of hops, wild oregano, chamomile, and cinnamon. The formula is exceedingly effective for chronic insomnia, as demonstrated by the following case history:

CASE HISTORY: Mr. I. is a long-term sufferer of insomnia, often having a hard time falling asleep, while also waking up frequently in the middle of the night. Thrashing and turning side-to-side, there was seemingly nothing that worked that eased him to sleep. He decided to try the full anti-insomnia spice complex consisting of extracts of hemp, wild oregano, hops, and chamomile, taking five drops at bedtime. He was astonished at the results, falling asleep virtually immediately after every use. It was a most astonishing result, and he was greatly relieved to finally be able to sleep well.

Treatment protocol

In the treatment of insomnia take the whole food extract of hemp plus wild oregano, five or more drops under the tongue at bedtime. Repeat as needed. For stubborn situations take the sleep aid complex of various sources of Beta-caryophyllene and cannabinoids, consisting of CO_2-extract hemp plus wild oregano, along with CO_2 extracts of chamomile, hops, and cinnamon: five or more drops at bedtime. Additionally, use the oil of wild oregano topically, rubbing it on the soles of the feet and the upper chest, also up-and-down the spine. If suffering from adrenal exhaustion, it helps to support such organs. This can be done by taking a specialized supplement for balancing the adrenal glands consisting of raw adrenal glandular material plus royal jelly and supportive herbs: two or more capsules at bedtime (see www.cassingram.com). Also, a salty snack at bedtime greatly aids in adrenal relaxation, thus causing the induction of sleep. Blood sugar imbalances secondary to adrenal exhaustion are a major cause of sleeplessness.

Sleep apnea

Regarding this condition as in some cases of insomnia the cannabinoids are effective. As reported in 2015, ABC-11, Raleigh-Durham, North Carolina, there is now a potentially FDA-approved anti-sleep apnea aid based on cannabis. Researchers are studying a cannabis-based pill for treating the condition. The treatment consists of the pill, along with a CPAP mask, which is worn overnight to aid in steady, regular breathing during sleep.

What a miserable way to attempt to fall asleep, that is with a mask on the face, a suffocating nightmare. Plus, it would have to be kept ultra-clean to prevent fungal infection. By rooting out the cause of sleep apnea it can be reversed without resorting to such measures. The major causes of this condition are hypothyroidism, poor cellular oxygen metabolism, B complex deficiency, magnesium deficiency, chronic fungal infection, sugar excess, GMO poisoning, and food intolerance. Parasitic infestation may also play a role, and surely infection by mold is frequently a major player.

The medication, though, used in the mask treatment is the same as is the standard in modern medicine: a synthetic, patented drug, known as Dronabinol, the same one used to treat chemotherapy-induced nausea. Even so, the investigators have found that the drug helps keep airways open during sleep. No doubt, the whole crude extract is far more effective in this regard: without any risk of side effects. Too, it must be realized that the whole crude extract is fortified with raw, wild oregano, which is a most astoundingly powerful agent for upper airways, that is bronchial tube health. Wild oregano alone is highly effective in the reversal of this condition. The oil should surely be used but also the juice or aromatic essence. This essence is a dense source of molecular oxygen. One way to determine if a person is deficient in such oxygen is to look at the fingernail beds, particularly the first three fingers. If there is a lack of half moons on these fingers or if they are barely visible, then, this is a sign of cellular oxygen deficiency. That deficiency is often corrected through the intake of rich sources of B complex. However, in terms of herbal or natural medicines the juice of wild oregano and wild chaga are supreme.

Treatment protocol

To reverse sleep apnea take the wild oregano-hemp combination, five or more drops under the tongue at bedtime or one capsule as an alternative. Also, rub oil of wild oregano on the chest area upon retiring. Additionally, consume the juice of wild oregano, a half ounce twice daily. For extreme cases take an ounce of this juice/essence right at bedtime. For stubborn situations also take the sleep aid complex of various sources of Beta-caryophyllene and cannabinoids, consisting of CO_2-extract of hemp plus wild oregano, along with extracts of chamomile, basil, and cinnamon: five or more drops at bedtime. Additionally, consume wild chaga tea, ideally the type with wild birch and larch bark (that is ChagaBlack), two cups or more daily. Consume also whole food B complex powder made from rice bran, rice germ, and torula yeast, two tablespoonfuls daily. Supporting the thyroid gland also aids in the reversal of this condition. Support this function with a high quality natural supplement aimed at enhancing the function of this gland. Also, consume foods naturally rich in iodine such as seafood, wild fish, grass-fed beef, eggs, dulse, and kelp. Strictly avoid the consumption of refined sugar. Wheat or gluten may be an issue. A trial can be made on a gluten-free diet, as gluten restriction may aid in reversing this condition.

Heart and circulatory disease

Because of their actions on key receptor sites, cannabinoids do far more than merely balance brain and nerve function. For instance, they also have direct actions on the circulatory tree, both the heart and arterial system. It was Z. Jarai and his group publishing in the *Proceedings of the National Academy of Sciences* who made the connection. Here, it was discovered that cannabinoids act on the entire cardiovascular system in a highly positive way. Through their interaction with CB2 receptors they cause dilation of blood vessels thereby improving the delivery of blood to the tissues, in this case in regard to the gut blood vessels, known as mesenteric circulation. This enhanced blood flow is known as increased perfusion. Increased perfusion of blood to the gut is highly beneficial to the heart, because it preserves the blood flow to this organ. Digestion draws up to 65% of all blood from the body, often leaving the heart starved for oxygen.

Yet, cannabinoids also have direct, positive actions on the heart. Once again, this is a result of the relaxant effects mediated by CB2 receptor activation. The heart itself is largely a neurological organ and operates through the firing of nerve impulses. In this regard people have heart attacks when they are under emotional stress, for instance, when hurt, angry, frustrated, anxiety-ridden, and/or depressed. It happens often when people take events that surround them, literally "to heart." All these emotions directly affect the autonomic nervous system, leading to a depression and/or excessive excitation of cardiac function.

Emotions are often difficult to control. Excessive worry can weaken the heart, ultimately resulting in mild-to-moderate heart attacks. If combined with anger, repressed rage, or extreme psychic stress, a fulminant heart attack may occur, which could result in fatality. The heart is a nerve-based organ and can readily store derogatory impulses. There is need to gain a handle on the emotions, to set them into balance, all in order to be in optimal cardiovascular health. Therefore, it is a good policy to take a high-quality hemp CO_2 extract on a regular basis, if for no other reason than cardioprotection.

Moreover, wild oregano is good for the heart. In antiquity it was used for both heart failure and angina. In fact, oil of wild oregano is one of the most potent anti-angina agents known. Effectively, it helps maintain the heart as an efficient pump. This is why the hemp and wild oregano should always be taken together.

A sense of calm within the nervous system is the antithesis of the typical emotional stress seen in cardiac cases. That is what the intake of crude, whole food hemp extract achieves. This is true of not only the CO_2 component but also the cold-pressed oil, hempseed protein, and the seed itself. The latter two foods have the added benefit of being dense sources of magnesium, much needed by the heart muscle for optimal function. An extreme deficiency of this mineral is a precursor to heart attacks, strokes, and hypertension.

Notes P. Pacher in *Cardiovascular Pharmacology of Cannabinoids* the hemp active ingredients exert their effects through a relaxation of the heart and arterial tree. This leads to an actual increase in blood flow to the tissues. Now, it is not difficult to consider the immense value of the hemp compounds in one of the major cardiovascular syndromes: hypertension. In fact, says Pacher, cannabinoids "are considered novel antihypertensive agents." Moreover, they are also effective for treating and even reversing myocardial ischemia, he makes clear, especially if combined with extract of wild oregano. In fact, the wild oregano-hemp oil complex as sublingual drops is ideal for the treatment of angina and other cardiac ischemic syndromes.

Other investigators have determined that the daily intake of cannabinoids can affect the heart rate, largely in a positive way. This is by decreasing it, which can be of value in certain heart conditions manifested by a racing heart or heart rhythm disturbances. The fact is a hemp oil-wild oregano oil combination is an ideal therapy for any condition associated with a rapid heart rate, including excessively high resting heart rate, atrial fibrillation, palpitations, and supraventricular tachycardia. In contrast, the psychoactive type of cannabis, rich in THC, tends to do the opposite, causing a rise in heart rate, while also causing in some users heart rhythm disturbances. Often, it causes palpitations to the extreme, where the heart feels like it is going to explode: a most unpleasant sensation, indeed. This is due to an overload of the heart's CB1 receptor sites by high-THC marijuana, along with toxicity to the organ from smoking-induced carbon monoxide.

Today, there is an epidemic of coronary artery disease. Much of this is associated with restriction in blood flow as a result of constriction of the coronary arteries. Hemp has a positive effect in this regard. As published in the *Journal of Cardiovascular Pharmacology* cannabinoids were found to exert powerful effects in rats with constricted coronary arteries. Here, it was discovered that as a result of CB1 and CB2 receptor activation within heart tissue there was both coronary vasodilation, that is increased perfusion or blood flow, along with an increased pumping power of the heart muscle. Apparently, a modest activation of the CB1 receptors is not necessarily harmful and may actually aid in cardiac function. As would be expected, regarding marijuana, heart-related symptoms are most common with excessive or heavy use. This is in part due to the toxicity of smoke residues, which include the cardiac poison carbon monoxide. Rare or occasional use will not likely cause cardiac sequelae.

Treatment protocol

In the treatment of heart disease it is ideal to use not merely CBD oil but, rather, the full cannabinoid complex as an unrefined CO_2 extract. Take the raw hemp-wild oregano complex, five drops twice daily, increasing the dose if emotional distress is extreme. Or, take it as gelcaps, one twice daily. Also, consume organic, cold-pressed hempseed oil, two tablespoons daily, along with a high-quality hempseed-based protein powder, ideally fortified with sprouted brown rice protein powder, two tablespoons daily. Sprinkle hemp seeds on all food. Stick to a low carbohydrate diet, and strictly avoid the consumption of refined sugar as well as alcohol. For people with hypertension it would also be ideal to consume oil of black seed, two or more tablespoonsful daily, along with wild chaga-birch bark tea, two cups daily. As a rich source of raw cannabinoids and natural magnesium drink also the raw, unprocessed, whole hemp juice combined with spice oil antioxidants, an ounce or more daily. For a weak heart or enlarged heart thyroid assessment is necessary. Blood tests are helpful, but a more thorough approach is self-testing for the hormone type (see *The Body Shape Diet*, Knowledge House Publishers, same author).

Glaucoma

There is significant evidence indicating the efficacy of hemp extract in this potentially disastrous condition. The fact is world-wide glaucoma is one of the leading causes of blindness. It is caused by an increase in fluid pressure within the eye. This increased pressure can cause a cut-off of blood supply to the retinal cells, including the so-called retinal ganglion cells, leading to their death and, therefore, blindness. Even the pressure alone can do this, leading to cell death through mechanical destruction. Research has also determined a chemical cause for cell death, which is the accumulation of the toxin, peroxynitrite, a lipid peroxide.

The hemp extract use is not new. It was first recorded in the 27th century B.C. by the Chinese.

In modern medicine the connection between marijuana and glaucoma was first reported in smokers, who benefitted from a 3 to 4 hour reduction in intraocular pressure after smoking. However, further research determined that no long-term benefit could be gained through this method of administration, that is in most cases the reduction could not be sustained.

The ideal mode of administration is topical application and/or sublingual drops. Regarding sublingual drops a study published in the *Journal of Glaucoma* found that at a modest dose, five mg of cannabinoid, in this case, synthetic THC, there was a temporary reduction in intraocular pressure. In another study A.B. El-Remessy and his group found that in a glaucoma model both THC and cannabidiol protected through topical administration retinal neurons from degenerating. The mechanism of action was determined. The cannabinoids blocked oxidative damage, specifically the toxicity of a free radical known as peroxynitrite. In other words, they halted lipid peroxidation. This led the investigators to deem cannabinoids to be a "novel topical therapy for the treatment of glaucoma." Yet, wild oregano itself is a far more potent intracellular antioxidant than cannabinoids alone. Thus, a combination of these two natural complexes is ideal for reversing this condition.

Additionally, regarding the synthetics pure THC is not the safest way to treat this disease, whether internally or topically. As demonstrated in *Explemental Eye Research*, 1984, chronic use of the drug is associated with side effects, including cataract-like lesions, swelling and redness, and generalized irritation. In test animals, in this case cats, the cataracts developed within a mere five days. Therefore, in eye diseases only the whole food form of cannabinoids should be used, ideally fortified with wild oregano extract. There is also the wild oregano-hemp plus wild nettle oil cream, which can be applied gently to the upper eyelids or below the eyes (slight, temporary burning sensation may occur).

Treatment protocol

To properly treat this condition all types of whole food hemp sources should be consumed: the raw, organic CO_2 extract, the whole food, raw protein powder, and the cold-pressed seed oil. Additionally, for optimal results wild oregano extracts should be consumed, as glaucoma can be related to both parasitic and fungal infection. Take the whole food, raw hemp-wild oregano complex, five or more drops under the tongue twice daily. Additionally, consume two tablespoons of hempseed protein powder twice daily, along with one tablespoon of cold-pressed hempseed oil twice daily. Additionally, take the oil of wild oregano, edible type, wild-source, three drops under the tongue twice daily, as well as wild, raw greens extract made from wild, raw dandelion, burdock, and nettles as sublingual drops, 40 drops under the tongue twice daily. Also, consume the raw, unprocessed hemp greens extract combined with spice oil antioxidants, one half ounce or more daily. Rub the wild oregano-hemp-wild nettle cream below the eyes and gently apply on top of the upper eyelids (avoid directly putting into the eyes); slight, temporary burning sensation is normal; this may also help with floaters. Strictly avoid the consumption of alcohol and refined sugar as well as caffeine and chocolate. Note: wild chaga-birch bark tea aids in the reversal of this condition; drink two or more cups daily.

Chronic pain syndromes

It makes sense that cannabinoid-rich complexes, such as extracts of hemp, wild oregano, black pepper, wild sage, clove, and basil, would help modulate chronic pain. It is all about CB2 receptor site activation.

Pathological pain requires heavy-duty action. As an alternative to potential noxious drugs hemp extract plays a key role. It is particularly valuable for the treatment of pain which is unresponsive to orthodox treatments. As a result of their action on receptor sites and the ability of these compounds to modulate neurotransmitter formation cannabinoid-rich complexes are effective for virtually all pain syndromes. They can be used solely or in conjuction with standard treatment. For optimal results they can be used with wild oregano therapy, using oil of wild oregano topically and taking the whole, crude herb in capsule form internally.

In one case a person reported a most astounding improvement in his daughter, a sufferer of the connective tissue disease, Ehlers-Danlos syndrome. The condition, manifested by hyper-mobility, leads to significant pain, often in the knee joints. The treatment was applied to a four year-old, who complained of "knees paining inside." After two weeks of taking modest doses, a few drops every morning, the pain was eliminated. For the first time in her life she was fully mobile, running about and playing with her friends: pain-free.

The benefits versus chronic pain are to be expected. Cannabinoids are signaling agents, helping the body cope with stressors, and this includes pain and inflammation. In all chronic pain states the use of cannabinoids must be considered, even as an adjunct to medication. These substances are effective both internally and topically. Regarding the cannabinoids Beta-caryophyllene, in particular, is highly effective in the treatment of pain. In hemp extract as mentioned previously high-quality, raw extract may contain in the terpene fraction up to 50% caryophyllene by weight. The sophisticated wild oregano/hemp complex has a density of up to 60%, which is unmatched. With wild oregano oil and/or the CO_2 extract it is also high, up to 12%. Black pepper is exceptionally rich, with some forms measuring as high as 57% Beta-caryophyllene. Considerable amounts are also found in basil, rosemary, and sage as well as cloves. All such spices have a prolonged history as agents for pain and inflammation. In addition, cloves, rosemary, and wild oregano posess anesthetic-like actions, as does hemp. This is largely a consequence of the Beta-caryophyllene content.

There is no doubt about the efficacy of this complex. In fact, caryophyllene-rich herbs and spices, such as rosemary, sage, basil, cloves, oregano, cannabis, and more, have a long history in the use against pain syndromes and inflammatory diseases. The potency and power of the hemp-wild oregano components is demonstrated by the following case history:

CASE HISTORY: Ms. A. W. of Brookeland, Texas, has suffered polio and post-polio syndrome for all her life. For some five months she has taken the wild oregano-hemp complex. For the first time that she can recall she has benefited from "diminished pain" in her joints and has felt "fast relief." The wild oregano-hemp complex had a significant 'side effect,' which was to calm her down and make her feel naturally at ease, a feeling she never experienced prior.

Treatment protocol

In the treatment of chronic pain consume a hemp-wild oregano CO_2 extract complex, five or more drops under the tongue three times daily. Additionally, take oil of wild oregano, edible type, five drops twice daily, also using the oil vigorously as a topical rub. There may also be need to take antiinflammatory plant enzymes; take a bromelain-papain enzyme complex with antiinflammatory herbs, two capsules on an empty stomach twice daily. If the pain is within the nerve sheaths, consider wild, raw turmeric extract as sublingual drops, 20 drops twice daily. Furthermore, for extreme cases use also the specialized bone- and joint-building capsules consisting of wild, raw oregano, rosemary, and sage, along with raw New Zealand-source grass-fed bone extract, two or more capsules twice daily.

A rubbing oil is available made from caryophyllene-rich wild oregano, rosemary, and sage. This can be rubbed vigorously all over the body and is particularly effective against rheumatic joints: use as often as desired and take five drops under the tongue twice daily. Also, use a wild oregano-hemp-wild nettle oil-based cream with propolis and Canadian balsam, applying as often as needed. This is a highly effective therapy for any inflammation-related or pain syndrome.

Migraine headaches

There can be no doubt about the fact that the raw hemp-oregano oil combination is an effective treatment for migraines. These headaches are associated with defective neurological function as well as disruptions in the digestive processes. Often, they are provided by intolerances to certain foods and beverages. The intolerances lead to an inflammatory response which goes out of control, leading to migraines. Cannabinoids help modulate this, particularly the ubiquitous terpene Beta-caryophyllene. The compound is found in dense amounts in precisely those herbs and spices, wild oregano, wild rosemary, holy basil, and ginger, known to reverse migraine attacks.

Historically, cannabis has been a recorded treatment for migraine and other headaches. With its direct, powerful action on nerve centers and on reducing inflammation this is no surprise. Furthermore, cannabis is an analgesic and to some degree an anesthetic agent, so it will relieve headache pain. Yet, so has wild oregano oil, which was used by the ancient Greeks and Romans as a headache remedy. In fact, as sublingual drops oil of wild oregano alone, edible-type, high-mountain-source often obliterates this condition. That's why the combination of hemp with wild oregano is so potent, as demonstrated by the following case history:

CASE HISTORY: Ms. M. is a big fan of natural medicine who was attending a trade show. At that show she suffered a severe migraine headache. Her remedies were unsuccessful in relieving it. She was given the hemp-wild oregano complex, which she took as drops under the tongue, about 20 drops at a time. Within a mere half hour the headache was obliterated.

Additionally, wild, raw far northern-source greens, that is wild greens bitters, are an effective remedy against this condition. The wild, raw greens cleansing agent consists of extracts of raw, wild dandelion, burdock, and nettles. Taken sublingually, it is a highly effective anti-migraine agent, make no mistake about it.

Treatment protocol

The cannabinoids are a group of many different natural analgesics that prove invaluable in chronic pain syndromes, including migraines and other headache conditions. To treat headaches take the raw hemp-wild oregano complex, five or more drops under the tongue as often as necessary. Also, rub this complex on the forehead; it's rich in green pigments and may stain clothes and sheets. For extreme cases take edible oil of wild oregano (P73 blend), five drops under the tongue as often as necessary. Also, take the wild, raw greens cleansing agent, a half dropperful under the tongue as often as necessary as a therapeutic purge. Because of its cleansing powers and dense source of the muscle relaxant magnesium, the raw hemp greens extract may prove invaluable; take a half ounce once or twice daily. Additionally, avoid the consumption of the most noxious allergenic foods, as described in *Natural Cures for Headaches* (Knowledge House Publishers, same author), which include cheddar cheese, Swiss cheese, wheat, rye, cocoa, MSG, and NutraSweet.

Chronic lung and bronchial disorders

Regarding disorders of the lungs and bronchial tree, no doubt, cannabinoids are invaluable. Here, in their role as signaling agents they help create a balance in lung function. Yet another internal power of these compounds is their antiinflammatory capacity. There are also flavonoids in hemp which help ease irritation and inflammation along the bronchial linings. The cannabinoid receptor activators in hemp are also antitussive agents, which means they help eliminate irritating, chronic cough. This is in part by normalizing the flow of mucous. Additionally, in particular, hemp seed and hemp seed protein are dense sources of magnesium, as is the fresh-extracted juice, and this mineral is essential for lung function. The lung matter itself is dependent on a goodly supply of plant omega 6s and 3s, and these are sufficiently supplied by hempseed oil. Such plant oils are essential for the maintenance of the health of those crucial lung cells known as the alveoli, which are responsible for oxygen exchange. These oils also act as natural antiseptics, keeping the bronchial tubes free of germs.

Far more potent as a germicide is oil of wild oregano. It is a most vigorous remedy for lung conditions. In fact, no lung condition is a match for this potent, therapeutic oil:

CASE HISTORY: What could be more dire than COPD, a condition where a person can't even breathe? In medicine it is a virtual death sentence for the victim. A woman who had the condition for 20 years after reading the book *The Cure is in the Cupboard* (Knowledge House Publishers, same author, 20th Edition, Expanded and Revised) decided to avail herself of the oil. Having already used dozens of other natural or herbal remedies, largely to no avail, she held out little hope. By taking a large dose, 20 drops twice daily, she had a remarkable improvement: some 80% of her COPD symptoms were eradicated in a mere two weeks.

The combination of hemp-oregano oil is a most thorough, potent natural medicine for lung conditions. While the cannabinoids activate the signals necessary for lung cell balance, the wild oregano acts as a powerful germicide. The following protocol is useful for any lung condition, including chronic bronchitis, COPD, emphysema, pulmonary fibrosis, TB, and asthma:

Treatment protocol

To treat this condition take the hemp-wild oregano complex, five or more drops twice daily, increasing the dose, as needed. For extreme conditions use the super-strength variety, 10 or more drops twice daily. Take also the oil of wild oregano, five or more drops twice daily, along with the whole crude herb complex with *Rhus coriaria*, two capsules twice daily. For resistant conditions it may be necessary to take the multiple spice complex consisting of dessicated wild oregano and sage oils, along with cumin and cinnamon oils, one or two capsules twice daily as well as the juice of wild oregano, an ounce daily. Consume also spice-infused organic hempseed oil, two tablespoonfuls daily as a means for lung regeneration. In the case of tuberculosis the dosages of all such remedies must be doubled or tripled.

Fibromyalgia

Regarding various inflammatory disorders, such as fibromyalgia, the hemp-wild oregano therapy is a most potent therapy. This is related to the basis of this syndrome, since this condition is due largely to infection. The culprits include giardia, candida, mold, and viruses. In addition, Lyme infection, that is infection by spirochetes, is also a major causative factor.

The infections cause inflammation, which then leads to the symptoms of fibromyalgia. One of the other issues is leaky gut syndrome. This leads to muscular and joint pain, yet, once again, the cause is infestation. To reiterate mold and fungus are major causes of this syndrome. To cure the condition the molds and fungi must be purged from the body. Regardless, the wild oregano-hemp sublingual drops and/or capsules is the ideal therapy for reversing this condition. So is the malic acid- and Beta-caryophyllene-rich wild oregano/rhus capsules.

Treatment protocol

To treat this condition take the hemp-wild oregano complex, five to ten drops two or more times daily. For tough cases take the super-strength form, 10 or more drops three times daily. Also, take the whole, crude wild oregano complex, along with *Rhus coriaria*, the latter being rich in malic acid, two or more capsules twice daily. Additionally, take the juice of wild oregano, one ounce daily. For severe muscular pain use the bone-activating rubbing oil consisting of oils of wild oregano, sage, and rosemary, rubbing into any areas of severe discomfort and pain. To resolve the leaky gut syndrome take the healthy bacterial supplement, Ecologic 500, a teaspoonful of the powder in a glass of water at night.

Plantar fasciitis

In virtually all inflammatory conditions extract of hemp plays a role. The same is true of wild oregano oil. In one study conducted by Turkish investigators the oil demonstrated anti-pain and antiinflammatory powers nearly equal to non-steroidal antiinflammatory agents.

In this condition there is considerable inflammation in the tissues on the soles of the feet, notably the plantar fascia. Treatment involves consumption of the wild oregano/hemp complex, along with topical application of this oil and/or the super-strength oil of oregano. The wild oregano-hemp-wild nettles cream may also be used as a topical treatment.

Treatment protocol

To treat this condition take the hemp-wild oregano complex, five or more drops twice daily under the tongue, increasing the dose, as needed. Also use the oil mixture topically, rubbing on the soles of the feet and leaving it there, covered by socks. Repeat daily until the condition is resolved. Note: plantar fasciitis can be due to B complex deficiency, notably a deficit of pantothenic acid. To correct this take a whole food B complex supplement powder, avoiding the typical coal tar-based pills, two tablespoonsful twice daily.

Chapter Nine

Neurological Conditions Resolved

In terms of therapeutic value perhaps the greatest domain for the cannabinoids is neurological conditions. After all, these substances are signaling agents for nerve tissue. A deficiency in these substances results in a gross imbalance in nerve cell conduction. Moreover, it is the nerve tissue which exerts ultimate control over the internal organs. In this section the various neurological conditions, as well as psychiatric ones, that are responsive to hemp therapy are described. These conditions include those due to actual pathology, like infection and/or degeneration of brain tissue, along with conditions caused by chemical imbalances and nutritional deficiencies.

ALS (Lou Gehrig's disease)

This condition, represented by gross degeneration of brain tissue, is directly related to infectious disease. In ALS there is always an infectious component, where critical cells and organ systems of the brain are fully infested. This leads to cell death of the neurons. Once the brain matter degenerates, nerve impulses are impeded and/or halted. The muscles can no longer get their nourishment, and they degenerate. The person ultimately becomes an invalid with no muscle function, unable to move, swallow food, or even breathe normally, living on liquids transported through feeding tubes.

Like all conditions it is crucial to determine the cause in order to achieve the cure. Viruses are suspected, particularly echoviruses. Yet, it has been fully demonstrated that in this condition the brain is infected with other highly invasive germs, for instance, spirochetes, notably that terminally noxious agent, the Lyme spirochete *Borrelia burgdoferi.* Thus, tick bites may precede the onset of this disease. There is also a role played by septic meat, notably the type raised on feed tainted with animal matter. Mad cow syndrome, the human variant being known as Creutzfeldt-Jakob syndrome, is a very real cause of ALS. This is caused by an unknown legion of germs or germ-related elements, notably infective prions, which are introduced into cattle as a result of the disease-ridden feed. A high percentage of ALS victims have a history of the consumption of large amounts of commercial meat, particularly beef.

Toxicity also predominates as a key factor, notably overload of heavy metals and noxious chemicals. The chemicals that play the greatest role in the cause or aggravation of this disease are pesticides, herbicides, and fungicides. Furthermore, the metals cadmium and mercury greatly weaken the blood-brain barrier, increasing the toxicity of noxious chemicals and infectious agents.

In addition, there is the issue of vaccines, which directly contaminate the body with heavy metals, notably aluminum and mercury. Even more dire they are a major source of noxious pathogens, introduced through injection, which may readily infect the brain stem and other cranial organs, ultimately leading to degeneration. The flu shot, in particular, can provoke this condition.

Trauma may also play a role, like repeated assaults to the head from physical abuse, motorcycle accidents, sports injuries, falls, and car accidents. No matter what the ancillary causes, though, in virtually all cases there is an infectious role in this condition.

The cannabinoids and other compounds in wild oregano extract, including the phenolic compounds, are invaluable in the treatment of this condition. In one small trial of physically incompetent ALS victims two of the 16 treated had a dramatic improvement through the use of the juice of wild oregano, along with the dessicated multiple spice complex. The doses were small; otherwise, the results would have likely been more positive. Even so, in one case a complete cure was achieved, and the patient is still alive and well, no longer wheelchair-bound. In addition, no doubt, the various phytochemicals in hemp CO_2 extract, as well as the seed oil, are effective adjuncts against this condition. Never give up hope. If used aggressively and if the condition is caught soon enough, natural medicines can reverse this disease.

Treatment protocol

To treat this condition a hemp-wild oregano extract is essential. Take 20 or more drops of a super-strength form of hemp-wild oregano CO_2 extract two or more times daily. Also, consume the juice or essence of wild oregano, one ounce or more twice daily, along with the dessicated spice complex, two capsules twice daily. If swallowing is difficult, use the wild multiple spice drops, 20 or more drops twice daily. The aromatic essence of wild oregano, wild sage, wild rosemary, plus rose and orange blossom may prove invaluable, an ounce or two twice daily. The consumption of wild chaga-birch bark tea is advised, as well as the total body purging agent, an ounce daily. Also, consume high-quality organic, first-pressed hempseed oil infused with spice extracts, one ounce or more daily.

Parkinson's disease

There can be no doubt about it Parkinson's disease is directly associated with pathogenic invasion of the brain stem. Invasive agents include fungi, parasites, bacteria, and vaccine viruses. There are other key factors, such as mercury and lead toxicity, as well as chronic exposure to pesticides and herbicides. The chemical action of these deadly substances is to poison the nervous system. Such toxic chemicals weaken the immunity and structure of brain tissue, making it vulnerable to invasion. In such cases it is ideal to consume the total body purging agent made with wild, raw greens extracts, along with black seed oil, as a means of causing the removal of such neurologically corrupting poisons. Another key agent is to consume the organically produced, cold-pressed hemp leaf juice.

Vaccines are a major cause of Parkinson's disease. These injections contaminate the body with live germs capable of attacking the brain. In fact, these inoculations are often the primary factor in sudden onset Parkinson's disease, the flu vaccine being a major culprit.

The infectious agents must clearly be purged. This demonstrates the value of wild oregano in the treatment of this condition. For optimal results both the oil and the aromatic essence must be consumed. In this condition there is much need to normalize neurological function. Actions on the endocannabinoid system aids in such normalization. In many respects Parkinson's disease is a deficiency one, that is a deficiency of key neurological components known as neurotransmitters. Endocannabinoid receptor activators, such as the phytochemical extracts of hemp and wild oregano, help boost neurotransmitter synthesis and also prevent such substances from degenerating. These cannabinoid-rich plants also act as antioxidants, preventing the age-related destruction of brain tissue.

So-called CBD oil acts not only on the endocannabinoid receptors but also on those responsible for the synthesis of serotonin and adenosine, both of which are deficient in this disease. Yet, even more powerful is the crude, raw carbon dioxide-extracted hemp complex, the one with the full panorama of cannabinoids, as this acts as a broad-spectrum antioxidant for preserving brain tissue. Yet, its antioxidant powers is greatly boosted through the addition of wild, raw oregano extract, the most potent herbal antioxidant known.

Treatment protocol

To treat this condition take the hemp-wild oregano complex as sublingual drops, 10 drops under the tongue two or more times daily. For extreme cases use the super-strength form, 20 or more drops three times daily. Also, in the event of heavy metal overload or chemical toxicity take the total body purging agent, one ounce or more daily for at least one month. Consume also the juice of wild oregano, one ounce or more daily, along with the dessicated spice complex, two capsules twice daily. If swallowing is difficult or impossible, use the wild multiple spice drops, 20 drops twice daily. The aromatic essence of wild oregano, wild sage, wild rosemary, plus rose and orange blossom essence may prove invaluable, an ounce twice daily. The consumption of wild chaga-birch bark tea is advised, as well as the total body purging agent, an ounce daily.

Schizophrenia

There can be little doubt about the fact that this disorder is a cannabinoid deficiency syndrome. Immediately upon replenishing these substances the condition improves. The brain centers in schizophrenia are fully depleted of neurotransmitters as well as the cannabinoid signaling agents. This is why with hemp therapy improvement can be rapid, virtually overnight.

There are other factors to consider in this disease. These factors include the role of nutritional deficiency and also food intolerance. Common deficiencies include a deficit of B complex, magnesium, selenium, zinc, and essential fatty acids. Regarding food intolerance this is a predominant factor in this disease. Foods which are particularly noxious for schizophrenics include corn, rye, wheat, cheese, cocoa, and sugar. Regarding sugar, this is a primary addiction in schizophrenics. Furthermore, the majority of schizophrenics suffer from yeast/fungus overgrowth, largely because of excess sugar consumption. This demonstrates the powers of wild oregano oil, in particular, in purging this disease.

Treatment protocol

To treat this condition take the hemp-wild oregano complex as sublingual drops, 10 drops under the tongue two or more times daily. Also, in the event of heavy metal overload or chemical toxicity take the total body purging agent, one ounce or more daily for at least one month. Consume also the juice of wild oregano, one ounce or more daily, along with the aromatic essence of wild oregano, wild sage, wild rosemary, plus rose and orange blossom, one ounce twice daily. The latter is highly effective against reversing this disease and creates a sense of focus and calm unheard of in this condition. The consumption of wild chaga-birch bark tea is advised, two cups daily. Additionally, strictly curtail the consumption of refined sugar and corn products as well as wheat and rye.

Obsessive compulsive syndrome

Regarding this condition it is largely the result of poor dietary practices. These dietary practices lead to a depletion of adrenal reserve. The person can't cope and therefore develops the syndrome.

Is there truly any such condition? The fact is in all cases of obsessive compulsive syndrome exhaustion of the adrenal glands plays a key role. In most cases sugar addiction is also a primary element. Refined sugar rapidly exhausts adrenal reserves. In this regard it is not possible for a person to behave in a calm, collect manner with impaired adrenal function. Another key issue is candida infestation. The yeast produces toxins, such as candida toxin and formaldehyde, which greatly poison the nerves, leading to bizarre behaviors and/or the inability to cope.

Chocolate also exhausts the adrenal glands, especially the type made with sugar. The theobromines in cocoa can in some individuals greatly irritate the adrenal glands, leading to nervous agitation. The person compensates for the adrenal exhaustion by being compulsive in behavior patterns. In particular, such a person cannot handle potentially stressful or unexpected events, which explains to a degree the compulsiveness. Checking the car or home multiple times to see if it is locked or similar actions is merely a means of self-protection to avoid the stress of any catastrophes.

Treatment protocol

To treat this condition take the hemp-wild oregano complex, five drops under the tongue two or more times daily. Also, consume the aromatic essence of wild oregano, wild sage, wild rosemary, plus rose and orange blossom, one ounce twice daily. To boost adrenal function take the *Body Shape Diet* adrenal complex fortified with royal jelly and raw grass-fed adrenal glandular powder, two capsules twice daily. Be sure to increase the consumption of sea salt, as this bolsters adrenal function. To purge the candida take oil of wild oregano, five or more drops twice daily under the tongue or as a gelcap, one twice daily. Curtail the consumption of refined sugar and chocolate.

Stroke recovery

In stroke recovery it is essential to make every attempt to achieve brain cell regeneration. Raw CO_2-extracted hemp oil is premier in this regard. It is both neuroprotective and neuroregenerative. There have been a number of studies demonstrating its novel powers in inducing new brain cell growth, which is essential for stroke recovery. Wild oregano, too, has been found to aid stroke victims, often causing a partial or even full return of function. Among the types of wild oregano proven to be effective include the hydrosol or aromatic essence of wild oregano, the oil of wild oregano, edible type, and the CO_2 extract, as found in the hemp-wild oregano complex.

Science is only just beginning to understand how well-equipped the human brain is for adapting to serious assaults, including brain cell death. The brain is highly adaptable and is constantly seeking to self-repair in consequence of any insult. Known as brain plasticity, it means that this organ is continuously optimizing its functions, even when it is damaged or injured.

A stroke, for instance, can severely harm certain areas of the brain. Yet, a goodly portion of its functioning can be restored as neural connections are rewired in an attempt to compensate for the damage. Regarding hemp and/or wild oregano this restoration is largely dependent on that key active ingredient, caryophyllene. In particular, trans caryophyllene has been investigated for this effect, and the results have been promising with the substance improving oxygen delivery to brain cells. This is true even in the event of the reduction of blood flow to the brain or cerebral ischemia, which is the physiology of strokes. Essentially, the caryophyllenes help repair brain damage by preventing and/or reversing hypoxia, an incredible feat which relatively few natural substances can achieve.

Treatment protocol

To treat this condition take the hemp-wild oregano complex, ten or more drops under the tongue two or more times daily.

For extreme conditions increase the dose, 20 to 40 drops twice daily. Also, consume the aromatic essence of wild oregano, wild sage, wild rosemary, plus rose and orange blossom, one ounce twice daily. Drink also the juice of wild oregano, an ounce twice daily. In addition, consume the fatty wild salmon oil, rich in natural vitamins D and A, one tablespoonful daily. As well, consume spice oil-enhanced organic hempseed oil, two T. daily.

Autism

A pandemic condition, autism is largely a vaccine-induced corruption. The vaccines or, rather, inoculations induce chronic infections into the tissues, especially within the lymphatic tissue as well as the brain. It was the British internist Wakefield who made the lymphatic connection, finding hard proof of infestation by vaccine viruses, notably the viruses from the MMR shot. What Wakefield discovered was an intestinal infection by the viruses, notably in the lymphatic tissue of the gut known as the Peyer's Patches. For this he was mercilessly persecuted by the pharmaceutical cartel and its media handlers, with his medical licence ultimately being suspended. That demonstrates how powerful is his information and that he truly made the connection: that vaccines are the cause of this condition.

Neurologically, autism victims need support, as their brains have suffered damage from inoculation pathogens as well as noxious chemicals found in these injections. The greatest damage is done by the mercury, which is found in the vaccines in the form of thimerosal. Other destructive agents found in vaccines include squalene, aluminum salts,

MSG, aspartame, and formaldehyde, the latter being an extreme neurotoxin.

There can be no better treatment for autism than the combination of crude extract of hemp plus whole food, raw wild oregano extract. Both these raw herbal extracts act directly on those key brain tissue receptor sites, the endocannabinoid receptors. Beta-caryophyllene is particularly potent in activating the nerve-balancing receptor sites, which is found in both hemp and wild oregano extract in dense amounts. In this way a rather rapid action can be achieved in the reversal of this disease. In fact, in many respects the cannabinoids represent an outright cure for this condition. This is demonstrated by the following case report:

Senior Writer
June 3, 2015
Beth Greenfield

Controversial Cannabis Treatment Helps 9-Year-Old Boy Speak His First Words

Kalel Santiago, 9, who has autism, spoke his first words shortly after starting hemp-oil treatments.

Though Kalel Santiago of Puerto Rico is only 9 years old, he's already endured some adult-level struggles. At just 10 months, he was diagnosed with the rare childhood cancer neuroblastoma, and spent more than two years undergoing surgery, chemotherapy, and radiation treatments. Then came the next diagnosis: severe, non-verbal autism.

"While he was in the hospital, we noticed he didn't speak at all and had some behavior that wasn't right, like hand flapping, and walking on his toes," his father, Abiel

Gomez Santiago, tells Yahoo Parenting from the family's home in Aguada. "But we waited until he was 3 and cancer-free to look at his behavior." In just two days...

"He surprised us in school by saying the vowels, A-E-I-O-U. It was the first time ever," Abiel says. "You can't imagine the emotion we had, hearing Kalel's voice for the first time. It was amazing. The teacher recorded him and sent it to my wife and me and we said well, the only different thing we have been doing is using the CBD." Soon thereafter, he adds, Kalel started using consonants to connect his sounds. "He said, 'amo mi mama,' 'I love my mom,'" Abiel says. "I don't know how to thank (the makers of medicinal hemp extracts)."

Treatment protocol

To treat this condition take the hemp-wild oregano complex, five to ten drops or more under the tongue two or more times daily. The hemp-wild oregano combination may also be rubbed up-and-down the spine also on the bottom of the feet: warning - may stain the sheets and clothing. Also, consume the aromatic essence of wild oregano, wild sage, wild rosemary, plus rose and orange blossom, one ounce twice daily. Additionally, take the wild, raw greens flushing agent for gut detoxification, two dropperfuls twice daily. For brain regeneration and balance wild chaga should be consumed. This can be taken as a tea and also as wild, raw sublingual drops. For additional calming action take also the sleep aid complex of various sources of Beta-caryophyllene and cannabinoids consisting of CO_2-extract hemp plus wild oregano, along with extracts of chamomile, hops, and cinnamon: five or more drops at bedtime or whenever needed. For those taking CBD it is still advisable to consume the wild oregano-hemp complex as sublingual drops.

Chronic depression

Extract of hemp is one of the most sophisticated, effective treatments for this condition known. In fact, there is no better remedy for chronic depression than the cannabinoids. Even so, it must be realized that hemp extract is not the only source of these compounds. Other herbs/plants that have a vast history for the treatment of mental diseases, such as basil, wild oregano, wild rosemary, wild sage, and hops, are also dense sources of these compounds.

Yet, depression may be due to a variety of factors, including nutritional deficiency, stress, emotional imbalances, and even infectious disease. Regarding nutritional imbalances and/or deficiencies refined sugar plays a major role. A decided poison the substance greatly depletes nutrients from the body, including the B complex, as well as magnesium, causing imbalances in brain function. It also feeds candida yeast, which further complicates the dilemma.

Alcohol is another major cause of this condition, again by causing extreme nutritional imbalances. The substance aggressively depletes both the B complex and magnesium from the tissues. The consumption of hemp seeds and protein, a potent source of magnesium, is an essential way to correct this, while the green juice is a dense source of B complex. There is another element to this. The substance destroys the cells in the thinking part of the brain, the cerebral cortex, and, thus, depression is a common consequence. Blood sugar imbalances play a key role. These are common results from a high sugar diet or the intake of excessive amounts of starch. Additionally, excessive alcohol consumption can also lead to blood sugar disturbances.

Treatment protocol

In the treatment of depression activation of the cannabinoid receptor sites is a most potent therapy. Take the raw CO_2 hemp-wild oregano extract, five or more drops twice daily. In extreme cases use the super-strength form, five to ten drops twice daily, or take it as a gelcap, one two capsules twice daily. Also, consume a hempseed/sprouted brown rice protein powder complex, two or three tablespoonsful in juice or as a smoothie every morning. Use hemp seeds on foods or in cooking; take one or two tablespoonsful of organic, cold-pressed hempseed oil daily. If available, consume the raw, unprocessed, cold-pressed hemp juice, a half ounce or so daily.

Additionally, use the caryophyllene-rich aromatic hydrosol complex, the neurologically activating essences of wild oregano, sage, and rosemary, along with essences of rose and orange blossom, one or two tablespoonsful twice daily. Take also whole food B complex from rice bran, rice germ, and torula yeast, two tablespoonfuls daily. Eliminate refined sugar and alcohol. Gluten may also play a key role in depression and in most cases should also be eliminated. To purge the candida take the oil of wild oregano, edible type, wild-source, five or more drops twice daily. For eradication do this for at least two months, taking also probiotics, which should be taken at a separate time away from the wild oregano therapy.

Anxiety

A condition with a complexity of causes, these causes include nutritional deficiency, blood sugar disorders, hormonal imbalances, fungal overload, stress overload, and chronic viral infection. Nearly all cases of this condition are self-induced through emotional distress, essentially, wrong thinking. Sometimes, abuse can lead to it, like the tormenting from a noxious spouse.

There are surely dietary factors, for instance, the consumption of irritants to the nervous system such as refined sugar and alcohol. Both these substances cause damage and irritation to the adrenal glands, resulting in nervousness and anxiety. In all cases of anxiety refined sugar must be strictly avoided, as must be alcohol. In many cases it may be necessary to avoid stimulants, for instance, cocoa, cola bean, and caffeine, along with, surely, amphetamine-based drugs. As well, drug therapy, that is the use of medication to merely control or alter the symptoms, is never the answer and usually worsens the condition. Instead, the cause must be treated. One key factor is to resolve the nutritional deficiencies. These deficiencies are greatly aggravated as a result of the consumption of refined sugar. In this regard all sources of refined sugar must be purged from the diet.

The candida must also be purged. This can be achieved to a degree by the hemp-oregano complex but usually requires the additional intake of the antiseptic form of wild oregano, that is the oil of oregano. Regarding deficiencies, most crucially, the B complex must be replenished. This is best achieved through the intake of a whole food complex made from rice bran, rice germ, royal jelly, and torula yeast.

Even so, there can be no better remedy for anxiety and/or anxiety-neurosis than cannabinoid-rich complexes. Another powerful remedy is royal jelly, ideally combined with natural-source adrenal glandular powder from grass-fed cows. In the treatment of this condition both these natural medicines should be used.

Additionally, in many cases the use of caryophyllene-rich aromatic waters, that is the essence of wild oregano, sage, and rosemary, along with essences of rose and orange blossom, proves invaluable. This complex improves neurological function in the brain, leading to a sense of relaxation but also increased focus and memory powers. A combination of the aromatic essence complex plus the hemp-wild oregano formula is highly effective for medically resistant anxiety, as demonstrated by the following case history:

CASE HISTORY: Ms. T., a 45 year-old woman, has suffered from persistent anxiety for over a decade during which she was medicated with potent drugs. It is well established that withdrawal from anti-anxiety drugs, such as SSRIs, is a major challenge, fraught with potentially serious withdrawal symptoms. In an attempt to remove the drug she consumed the aromatic essence complex and hemp-wild oregano combination. Within one month she reduced the dosage of her medication by 80% without the slightest side-effects or withdrawal symptoms. This was possible because of the mood elevation effects achieved by the natural medicine therapy.

Treatment protocol

To treat anxiety-related conditions take the raw CO_2-extracted hemp-wild oregano complex, five or more drops under the tongue as often as necessary. Use it more aggressively if attempting to achieve drug withdrawal. Take it also a half hour or so before bedtime to relax. Additionally, consume the aromatic essence of neurologically balancing spice and flower extracts, one ounce or so twice daily. For B vitamin support take the whole food B complex powder, two tablespoonfuls every morning in juice, water, or a smoothie. Strictly avoid the consumption of refined sugar as well as wheat and rye. Also, consume a diet rich in natural fats and protein. Take a hempseed and sprouted brown rice protein powder, two tablespoonfuls in juice or a smoothie every morning. As well, in some cases of a high-level of irritability coffee and chocolate must be avoided.

Nervous agitation

Essentially a form of anxiety nervous agitation is listed, here, because it is often a form of anxiety that is not diagnosed. They are similar. However, in the agitation type the person often has structural components, obvious signs of irritability, like shaking of the arms, tapping of the feet, nervous tics or twitches, muscle spasms, and more. Tens of millions of people suffer from this. Rather than being diagnosed with any condition they just know they are nervous, and so do others around them.

Nervous agitation and obvious nervous behavior is merely a symptom of cannabinoid deficiency. Therefore, the condition greatly responds to the appropriate therapy. It may also be a deficiency, as in anxiety, of the B complex as well as certain minerals, like magnesium. There can also be protein deficiency. Plus, commonly, nervous agitation is due to blood sugar imbalances.

Complexes rich in caryophyllene are the most vigorous cure for this condition, as fully demonstrated by the following case history:

CASE HISTORY: Ms. M., a 75 year-old woman, suffered from a constant state of nervous agitation. In the health food business her daughter was deeply concerned about her, because she was about to undergo a medical procedure. This was the replacement of the battery in her pace-maker. Any event like this caused an increase in her agitation. One of her primary symptoms was virtually endless pacing in the morning, sometimes lasting as long as three hours. She rushed the package off to her: a bottle of the hemp-wild oregano extract, along with a bottle of a nervous system-balancing tonic, known as Neuroloft. This extract is a combination of aromatic essence of rose, orange blossom, rosemary, sage, and wild oregano.

That morning, there was a dramatic change. For the first time in her life that she could remember, the pacing was eliminated. It was an astounding result, and it prepared her perfectly for the upcoming medical procedure. Here is what her mother said, exactly, who is not inclined to take natural medicines: "What was that stuff you sent me? For the first time in years I had no pacing of any kind, and I felt unusually calm before the procedure."

Here is yet another example of not so much nervousness but, rather, of the power of wild oregano-hemp complexes to reverse stress-induced syndromes:

Mr. J. C. of Garfield, New Jersey, has been taking the wild oregano-hemp complex for a mere two months, going through two bottles. He reports that he "loves how it makes him feel with his (stress-induced) nervousness" and has seen "a huge change since taking it." He "felt very calm and relaxed," and he knows it is exclusively from this supplement and is recommending it to family and friends. Few if any other natural whole food supplements could achieve such a result.

Treatment protocol

To treat this condition take the hemp-wild oregano complex, five or more drops under the tongue as often as needed. Also, use the neurologically balancing aromatic essence complex, a tablespoon or more twice daily. Additionally, take a whole food B complex supplement, two tablespoonfuls daily, along with organic cold-pressed hempseed oil, two tablespoonfuls daily. Additionally, take a hempseed and sprouted brown rice protein powder, two tablespoonsful in juice or a smoothie every morning.

Multiple sclerosis

Seemingly, a mystery to modern medicine as it turns out it is not so mysterious after all. No doubt, multiple sclerosis, or MS, is directly associated with infection of the brain matter, which makes sense considering the nature of the lesions. These lesions are inflammatory or, rather, infectious plaques. These plaques are found on the nerve sheaths and other brain substance. Moreover, they are highly visible on MRIs and other brain scans. If the infection is purged, then, the patient can recover: often completely.

No one can deny the connection. In fact, the types of germs which can invade the brain are legion and include parasites, molds, yeasts, bacteria, and viruses. In this condition viruses play a predominant role, including a number of agents of the herpes family. The bacteria chlamydia may also be involved. A great culprit is the bacteria which causes Lyme, the spirochete *Borrelia burgdorferi*. It was microbiologist L. Mattman, Ph.D., who determined the role, finding nearly 100% of all cases infected, with active spirochete infection fully documented within brain tissue by special staining techniques.

There is also the issue of imbalances in neurotransmission. No doubt, in MS the function of the endocannabinoid system is disturbed. There are also, commonly, deficiencies of neurotransmitters such as serotonin and GABA. Regarding nutritional deficiencies these include deficits of magnesium, B complex, vitamin A, vitamin C, vitamin D, and vitamin E. In particular, vitamin E and C are needed to prevent oxidative damage in the brain. The antioxidant enzymes glutathione and superoxide may also be deficient. This demonstrates the need for nutrients or herbal medicines which boost the levels of these enzyme complexes. Selenium aids in glutathione synthesis, while intake of wild chaga can boost superoxide dismutase levels, as it is the densest source of this substance known.

The hemp-wild oregano complex is ideal for the treatment of this condition. Both these ingredients offer a wide range of actions which aid in the reversal of this disease. Both wild oregano and hemp boost the internal production of glutathione, a crucial enzyme for the prevention of brain cell degeneration.

Treatment protocol:

To treat this condition take the hemp-wild oregano complex as sublingual drops, 10 drops under the tongue two or more times daily. Also, in the event of heavy metal overload or chemical toxicity take the total body purging agent, one ounce or more daily for at least one month. Consume also the juice of wild oregano, one ounce or more daily, along with the dessicated spice complex, two capsules twice daily. If swallowing is difficult, use the oil of wild oregano, 20 drops two or three times daily. The oil under the tongue is a crucial treatment for this condition. Take also the organic, cold-pressed hempseed oil, one ounce daily. The aromatic essence of wild oregano, wild sage, wild rosemary, plus rose and orange blossom may prove invaluable, an ounce twice daily. The consumption of wild chaga-birch bark tea is advised, a well as the total body purging agent, an ounce daily.

Tourette's syndrome

Just what is Tourette's syndrome? It is a complex condition manifested by a variety of neurologically based symptoms, including visual perception imbalances, motor disabilities, learning deficits, mood disorders, lashing out behavior, ADD-like symptoms, panic disorder, social skills defects, and phobias as well as obsessions. There are also nervous tics and memory deficits in the majority of victims. The condition has all the hallmarks of a vaccine-induced disorder. Thus, it is no surprise that its major victims are children and young adolescents.

Affecting some one percent of the population it is not an easy syndrome to define or treat. Yet, cannabinoids are certainly one vehicle with promise in its reversal. Notes K. R. Muller-Vahle, M.D., of the Medical School of Hannover cannabis appears to minimize the symptoms of this disease, including the nervous tics and behavioral disorders. She even was able to get positive results in humans with high THC material without side effects. An earlier study showed the same. Published in 2003 in the *Journal of Clinical Psychiatry* the investigators found that the compound significantly reduced the tics, while the patients, adult Tourette's cases, suffered no untoward effects. In fact, the results were so encouraging that the researchers said that in drug therapy THC "should be tried" as an optional treatment for the general public.

Even so, there is no need to use THC to achieve this. It can be adequately done through the vigorous intake of the whole, raw CO_2 extract combined with the anti-Tourette's syndrome oil of wild oregano.

Treatment protocol

Both extract of hemp and wild oregano, rich in Beta-caryophyllene and cannabidiol, are ideal therapeutics for this condition. Take the hemp-wild oregano complex as sublingual drops, five or more drops twice daily. For extreme cases use the super-strength form, 10 or more drops twice daily. Use the super strength oil of oregano as a topical rub up and down the spinal column. Rub once or twice daily, plus rub on the bottoms of the feet and shins. As a means of detoxification take the wild, raw greens flushing agent, 40 or more drops twice daily. Also, use the neurologically balancing aromatic essence complex, a tablespoon or more twice daily. Additionally, take a whole food B complex supplement, two tablespoonfuls daily, along with organic cold-pressed hempseed oil, two tablespoonfuls daily. Do all therapies until the symptoms are completely resolved.

Brain damage

In some studies a most astounding effect of cannabinoid-rich hemp extracts has been seen. This is the regeneration of brain cells. In some studies it has been found that from hemp therapy new brain cells are formed.

The scientific data fully supports the claim for its regenerative powers. It is a most astounding issue, fully neglected for decades by modern medicine. What diabolical neglect it has proven to be, in fact, more than mere neglect: extreme resistance. Yet, here it is, fully available all over the world, the answer for nerve cell degeneration: for premature aging and damage to the brain. Notes Fernandez-Ruiz in his article published in *Neurotherapeutics* cannabinoids are precisely the answer to nerve cell damage or aging. It is these compounds which keep the nerve cells in their finest state of health, known as "homeostasis." Moreover, notes Fernandez-Ruiz, the "survival" of these cells is also cannabinoid-dependant.

The power of these molecules upon the nerve cells, including the cells of the brain and spinal cord, is truly impressive. The various actions of cannabinoids include preserving, repairing, and even rescuing neurons, that is those which are being damaged and intoxicated. It is not merely this. The cannabinoids, says this researcher, are capable of *replacing neurons,* a most incredible feat. To do this the cannabinoids clearly act upon the neurons directly, but so do they also act upon specialized cells known as neural progenitor cells, that is cells that function to generate new nerve cells.

Wild chaga may prove of value in the recovery from stroke. This is because of its rich content of cholesterol precursors known as inotodiol and lanosterol. It is cholesterol which in a modified state largely forms the coating of the neurons' all important coating, the myelin sheath. Moreover, every nerve cell in the body is structured based on this molecule, often bound to compounds such as choline and inositol. Chaga is also a dense source of rare trace minerals, such as rubidium, germanium, and cesium, which help activate neuronal function. Additionally, it is the world's top source of SOD, that antioxidant enzyme that is much needed to both prevent brain damage and also repair diseased or dysfunctional cells. The ideal type of wild chaga is the raw extract. In such a state the chaga sterols remain unaltered, which gives them their maximum biological activity and makes it easier for them to be transported through the blood-brain barrier. Raw chaga is available as sublingual drops, wild oregano-fortified capsules, and also as a cream (that is ChagaHeal and/or Chaga Face Cream).

Treatment protocol

To treat this condition take the hemp-wild oregano complex, 10 drops under the tongue two or more times daily. For extreme cases use the super-strength variety, which is three times more powerful, 10 to 20 drops three times daily. Also, consume the aromatic essence of wild oregano, wild sage, wild rosemary, plus rose and orange blossom, one ounce twice daily, along with the juice or essence of wild oregano, one ounce twice daily. Also, take raw chaga emulsion as sublingual drops, 3 dropperfuls twice daily and also apply the chaga cream on the face and soles of the feet as often as possible, also rubbing on the hands, shins, and up-and-down the spine. This will cause the transport of the key sterols and other therapeutic ingredients directly through the skin into the system.

Huntington's disease

Regarded as incurable this condition is manifested by progressive degeneration of brain tissue. It affects muscular contractions and leads to a decline in brain function and social capacities. There is significant research demonstrating the efficacy of hemp extracts in halting its progression. In one study published in the *Journal of Neuroscience Research* it was determined that both CBD and THC had positive effects on the rat model of this disease. The intake of these components stalled the disease progression, an effect thought to be due to these substances' antioxidant powers. It appeared that the cannabis-based medicine used in this study, the drug Sativex, acted as a neuroprotective agent, that is it prevented brain cell degeneration. Sativex is a cannabidiol-based drug. It has been fully established that this biological terpene induces regeneration of nerve cells. Yet, so does Beta-caryophyllene, among other key active ingredients in hemp and other green plants. Basil and wild oregano also have this power as a result of their rich content of the molecule, as does black pepper extract.

Treatment protocol

To treat this condition take the hemp-wild oregano complex, five drops under the tongue two or more times daily. For extreme cases use the super-strength form of this complex, 10 or more drops three times daily. Also, consume the aromatic essence of wild oregano, wild sage, wild rosemary, plus rose and orange blossom, one ounce twice daily. Additionally, consume the juice of wild oregano, also an excellent source of cannabinoids, an ounce twice daily; take as well cold-pressed organic hempseed oil, two tablespoonfuls daily.

Spinal disorders and pain

Regarding disorders of the spine and spinal column cannabinoid-rich hemp extracts are ideal. The same is true of wild oregano, as they both operate through similar mechanisms. The spinal column is an end-organ for cannabinoid activity. Readily, this region becomes dysfunctional in the event of defects in cannabinoid metabolism. Beta-caryophyllene, itself a cannabinoid, exerts profound influence over the health of the spinal

168 The Cannabis Cure

column and its nerves. Examples of spinal disorders which may respond to cannabinoid-caryophyllene therapy include spinal stenosis, chronic spinal infection, post-meningitis syndrome, kyphosis, scoliosis, Lyme inflammation syndrome, and ankylosing spondylitis. Additionally, the cannabinoids as signaling agents play a most crucial role, helping to create balance in the nerves of the spine, while aiding in the curbing of inflammation. Note: Spinal pain and inflammation can result from disease in the teeth such as abscesses and/or septic root canals. If this is the case, treat the teeth and gum areas with super-strength oil of oregano applied topically, along with the hemp-wild oregano complex. Virtually all spinal disorders respond to the hemp-wild oregano therapeutic regimen.

Treatment protocol

To treat imbalances in spinal health take the hemp-wild oregano complex, five to 10 drops twice daily. In extreme cases take the super-strength form, 10 to 20 or more drops two or more times daily. Consume also the juice of wild oregano, one ounce daily. As a spinal rub use the wild oregano oil. Another option is to rub the spinal column with the bone-activating rubbing oil. The hemp-wild oregano-wild nettle cream can also be used as a spinal rub. Also, drink the juice of wild oregano, one ounce twice daily. The hemp-wild oregano-wild nettle cream can also be used as a spinal rub.

Suicidal ideation and suicide

Is drug-induced suicide preventable? Is it even reversible when it is about to be enacted? In both cases the answer is a decided "Yes." That's because the condition is largely a chemical imbalance. Moreover, in most cases people who commit this act do so while on mood-altering drugs. Pharmaceutical drugs are the worst offenders, followed by recreational ones.

The activation of CB2 receptor sites is a key defense against suicide. This activation serves to induce a state of calm in the brain, largely through enhanced inter-neuron signaling. This is not the case with the hallucinogenic form, the type bred for its addictive powers, which can overpower the nervous system, accentuating suicidal thoughts. This demonstrates the noxious nature of marijuana breeding, that is the altering of the plant to cause it to be an intoxicant or to increase dramatically its hallucinogenic properties. People do this for only one purpose. It is to sell it for great profit. Yet, what are the consequences of this gross manipulation and greedy capitalism? In some cases the consequences are fatalities, including the incredibly destructive act of suicide, in this case of a young US Army veteran, Andy Zorn, as reported in the *Daily Courier*:

> He downplayed the mental toll of his overseas tour, and seemed to be adjusting to civilian life. Working part-time as an auto mechanic and studying for his degree, Zorn seemed happy. He was partying with friends, *experimenting with alcohol and marijuana* that he had first tried as a teenager.
>
> No one suspected anything out of the ordinary; indeed, he counseled friends struggling with addictions.
>
> Yet, Zorn's life trajectory was off kilter. He suffered from bouts of depression, started struggling in school and work, and his supposed recreational marijuana use became a secret shame. He was an addict.

On March 1, 2014, Zorn hanged himself; his suicide note blamed marijuana.

"Marijuana killed my soul + ruined my brain,' said Zorn's final message.

Surely, in addition to the over-use of marijuana post-traumatic stress syndrome played a role, here. Yet, how could a key role for the drug not be suspected in Zorn's case? According to his mother, Sally Schindel, under the influence of marijuana he became dysfunctional and was unable to complete common tasks. Despite being pro-medicinal hemp Schindel is now an activist against the legalization of pot, Andy Zorn became categorically dependent on the drug, which he was largely secretively smoking, spending all that he had on the habit: some $80,000-plus. Obviously, then, pot smoking did play a role in destabilizing him, which ultimately led to his untimely demise.

Does all this give pot a bad rap? That is irrelevant. All dangerous intoxicants must be exposed. No doubt, there is some justification in screaming bias and excesses. For instance, the punishment levelled against pot smokers is draconian. Yet, this doesn't take away from the fact that the consumption of hallucinogenic pot, whether through smoking, vaping, or ingestion, is simply not a good idea.

It seems that marijuana is more poisonous in this regard for early users. According to a study conducted by M. Lynskey and his group use of the drug before age 17 is associated with 3.5 times more attempted suicide than those who start smoking later in life. Marijuana numbs the senses. Thus, it clearly increases the risks for the potential of self-harm.

This is not the only death in recent times due to the drug. In Colorado three deaths have now been reported directly in consequence of marijuana intake. The latest case involved a 23 year-old, Luke Goodman, who killed himself through a self-inflicted gunshot wound. Said his mother, Kim Goodman, the death was a consequence of a "complete reaction to...drugs."

Goodman had according to an eyewitness eaten a number of the marijuana edibles, became agitated, grabbed the family gun, and then shot himself. No one should consume marijuana edibles made with high THC material, whether in reasonable amounts or large quanity.

The issue is the lax attitude toward pot. Few people are completely lax about, for instance, hard liquor. Drinkers know it is poisonous, and so do those who dispense it. With youths upon experimentation they may not realize the danger from edible pot products and, thus, have no means to prepare themselves for untoward consequences. Regardless, these are real deaths caused by a hallucinogenic substance. No such deaths should be taken lightly.

There can be no doubt that the cause of his death was the drug. Perhaps an even more glaring case involves a 19 year-old, Mr. L. Thamba Pongi. The youth specifically traveled with friends to Denver to experience marijuana edibles. Contrary to the clerk's advice he ate the entire edible instead of the suggested portion, in this case a THC-laced cookie. In the period after consumption of the poisonous cookie he acted erratically and violently, then some two hours later killed himself by jumping from the hotel's fourth-story window. It was the first time he ever used marijuana in any form.

In this case the tie to the drug was absolute, with high levels of THC and its metabolites being found upon autopsy, while there was no evidence of intoxication from any other drug, including alcohol. It was as if the edible was laced with a concentrated or synthetic form of the intoxicant. No wonder it overpowered his system. The deadly cookie contained some 65 mg of the highly biologically active THC or 10 mg per serving.

Surely, some people are more vulnerable to self-destructive acts than others. How depressed is the individual? What is going on in the depths of the person's spirit? It's also a matter of internal chemistry. What is the individual's nutritional status? Is such a one deficient in those mood-controlling substances, the B vitamins? Is there an excess of sugar in the diet, which causes nervous system irritability? Then, clearly, if the physiological and nutritional status is awry and then the individual consumes hallucinogens the consequences are surely unpredictable. In Mr. Zorn's case the use of both alcohol and marijuana proved ultra-dangerous. The marijuana apparently pushed him over the edge. His body proved unusually vulnerable, as did his psychic state.

Treatment protocol

To treat this condition take the hemp-wild oregano complex, five drops under the tongue two or more times daily. For extreme cases increase the amount, 10 or more drops as often as needed. Also, consume the aromatic essence of wild oregano, wild sage, wild rosemary, plus rose and orange blossom, one ounce twice daily. Wild chaga-birch bark tea also aids in detoxification; drink two cups daily. Wild, raw cranberry extract and wild, raw triple greens extract; take them as sublingual drops as part of the protocol in the event of substance abuse. To stabilize blood sugar and adrenal function take a royal jelly complex with wild rosemary and sage, two capsules twice daily. Correct all B vitamin deficiencies by taking a whole food B vitamin powder made from rice bran, rice germ, torula yeast, and royal jelly, two tablespoonsful twice daily. Strictly avoid the consumption of refined sugar, alcoholic beverages, noxious prescription drugs, pot, and corn products.

Chapter Ten

Digestive Disorders and More

The digestive system is a most crucial organ complex. For optimal health it must function in a balanced, orderly state. If it is disrupted, health throughout the entire body is disturbed. It is in some respects the most metabolically active, and demanding, element of the body. Upon eating, some 60% of all blood in the body is drawn to the gut. That demonstrates how truly influential is this system.

There is much need to keep the gut organ systems in balance, that is for the maintenance of optimal health. Regarding disorders of the digestive system raw, crude hemp extract plays a vast role. So do other top sources of cannabinoids such as wild oregano, wild rosemary, cloves, cinnamon, black pepper, and basil. The digestive system is a primary recipient of cannabinoid activity through strategically placed receptor sites. These receptor sites are found in all digestive organs and also in the immune system of the gut, the Peyer's Patches of the small intestine. Regardless, it has been long known; all caryophyllene-rich spices and herbs, for instance, basil, wild oregano, cumin, fennel, cloves, and black pepper, are digestive aids. The same is true of medicinal hemp, which has long been used for digestive disorders. One of the key reasons extract of hemp and the various spice concentrates are so crucial for gut health relates to inflammation. The hemp- and spice-based cannabinoids help modulate inflammation, a major issue in stomach and intestinal disorders as well as disorders of the liver and pancreas.

Inflammatory bowel disease

Caryophyllene helps with inflammation throughout the body, including the bowels. In this regard it is extremely beneficial in the treatment of inflammatory bowel disease. All inflammation-based bowel disorders respond to caryophyllene therapy. This includes spastic colon, irritable bowel syndrome, Crohn's disease, and ulcerative colitis. As well, extract of wild oregano, along with the whole, crude herb itself, is a potent therapy for these conditions.

Treatment protocol

To treat this condition take the oil of wild oregano-hemp oil complex, 5 or more drops under the tongue twice daily. For extreme conditions use the super-strength form, which is three times stronger, 10 or more drops twice daily. Also, take the crude wild oregano-*Rhus coriaria* complex, two or more capsules twice daily. Consume plenty of sources of probiotics, but beware of food intolerance such as reactivity to commercial milk products, wheat, rye, tea, coffee, and chocolate. Take a probiotic based on the strain, Ecologic 500. Also, consume a wild greens flushing agent based on raw, wild dandelion, burdock, and nettle, 40 drops twice daily.

Liver disease

The role of cannabinoids in the treatment of liver disorders is immense. The organ contains endocannabinoid receptors to receive dietary cannabinoids. The body makes these cannabinoids from fatty molecules, so it can regulate bodily functions, including the virtually endless roles played by this organ. Healthy detoxification, protein synthesis, bile production, and digestion are dependent upon sound cannabinoid function within liver tissue.

Yet, despite the diversity of its functions, rapidly, the liver can be overwhelmed with toxicity. To keep its regulatory function in optimal balance it is crucial to consume cannabinoid-rich foods and supplements. The cannabinoids keep liver cell function operating at the most optimal, thorough level possible—and such optimal function is nowhere needed more than in this organ. Conditions in this organ for which the cannabinoids may prove effective include generalized liver congestion, fatty liver, hepatitis, Gilbert's disease, and cirrhosis.

Curiously, in cirrhosis cells have an unusually high concentration of CB2 receptors. Yet, these receptors are largely absent in people who do not have the disease. It is thus believed that the endocannabinoids are playing a direct role in this condition, notably in the attempt to reverse it. Regarding the diseased cells, which are fibrotic, the body regards them as corrupt and seeks to purge them and/or inhibit their growth, an action achieved by the CB2-binding cannabinoids. In the liver the activation of these receptors leads to a reduction in fibrosis and also a boost in blood perfusion in the organ. Plus, antagonism to the liver's CB1 receptors turns out to be a positive element, as this stalls ascites, while impeding the progression of liver cell scar formation. Even so, there is no evidence that marijuana causes scarring of the liver. This is caused largely by alcohol as well as prescription drugs. Despite this, crude, whole food hemp extract is far more aggressive in reversing severe liver disease than marijuana smoke alone. This is particlarly true when it is combined with wild oregano oil, a most potent remedy for liver disorders.

Treatment protocol

For liver disease take ten drops of the hemp-wild oregano complex twice daily. For extreme cases use the super-strength form, up to 20 drops three times daily. Also consume organic hempseed oil, one tablespoonful daily. Take an organic, raw hempseed-based protein powder, two tablespoonfuls twice daily. Additionally, use a total body purging agent consisting of oils of black seed, extra virgin olive oil, wild sage oil, wild bay leaf oil, cumin oil, and fennel oil, along with wild, raw greens, an ounce or more daily. Avoid the intake of refined sugar, which is a potent liver poison. Also, categorically avoid the intake of alcoholic beverages, the primary cause of destructive liver disease.

Diabetes

Edible, whole food hemp extract is one of many effective natural remedies against this condition. Clearly, such an extract has significant, positive effects on the blood sugar mechanism. So do a litany of spices, also rich in cannabinoids such as cinnamon, allspice, cloves, basil, and wild oregano. In fact, spices are among the most potent blood sugar regulating substances known.

Regarding marijuana, it is spice-like. A study in Hadassah University Hospital, Jerusalem, determined that in diabetic mice cannabidiol "arrested the onset" of the disease, dropping the incidence of the disease by over 50%. This was regarding autoimmune diabetes, one of the most severe types, in fact, the one seen in the seemingly incurable Type 1 diabetes.

The cannabinoids are also effective against many of the side effects of this condition, notably diabetic neuropathy. Topical creams containing the oil have been found to aid in the reversal of diabetic numbness and tingling as well as restless leg syndrome. Moreover, cannabidiol acts also on the blood vessels of the eye and may aid in the prevention of diabetic blindness. Ultimately, the cannabinoids are attempting to regulate the body at all levels in this disease, preventing further degeneration.

Impaired regulation is the ultimate cause of diabetes. In fact, all the mechanisms involved in normalization are in disarray. Consider fat metabolism. Disrupted regulation of lipids is one of the key factors that leads to diabetes and its complications. A 2013 study demonstrated that caryophyllene aids in the regulation of lipids and may thus impede the progression of this disease and also act in prevention. It is known that a high spice consumption decreases the risks for this disease. In fact, massive, daily intake of the caryophyllenes is surely a means for diabetes prevention.

For reversing this disease the diet must be thoroughly addressed. All forms of refined sugar must be purged. In some instances gluten is an issue, as is the protein of cow's milk, casein. Additionally, the artificial sweetener aspartame is a potent pancreatic poison and must be eliminated from the diet. The intake of Beta-caryophyllene-rich spices, such as black pepper, cloves, cinnamon, cumin, rosemary, sage, thyme, Italian parsley, and wild oregano, should be considerable. For more information about the reversal of this disease through diet see *Natural Cures for Diabetes* (Knowledge House Publishers, same author).

Treatment protocol

To treat this condition take the hemp-wild oregano complex, 10 drops twice daily or for even more aggressive control, 10 drops with each meal. Also, take the essence of juice of wild oregano, one ounce or more daily. For nerve pain and other related symptoms use a hemp-wild oregano-based cream with Canadian balsam, propolis, nettle oil, used topically, as needed. Additionally, add powdered cinnamon to the daily regimen, a tsp. twice daily, or use the CO_2 extract, Cinnamol, as sublingual drops, 10 or more drops with each meal. Also take a whole food type of cumin oil, 10 drops twice daily.

Nausea and vomiting

Two of the main indicators for the use of medical marijuana are nausea and vomiting, especially when associated with chemotherapy. Both marijuana smoke and the drug isolates are effective in this regard, although excess smoking can act in an opposite fashion, causing cramps, nausea, and vomiting. Even more effective is the crude, raw extract combined with wild oregano. Both hemp and wild oregano have calming actions on the gut.

What's more, consider a common cause of these symptoms: infection. For instance, with infections of the liver nausea is a common consequence, particularly in the event of parasitic infestation. For the nausea, cramps, and vomiting to be halted the infection must be purged. This is why the wild oregano-hemp combination is more effective than merely CBD or cannabinoids alone. Regarding infestations of stomach and intestines there is, commonly, cramps but also nausea and vomiting. There can also be inflammatory causes of these symptoms as well as allergic reactions. In all instances the hemp-wild oregano complex proves effective.

Treatment protocol

To treat this condition take five drops of the hemp-wild oregano oil complex and hold it under the tongue as long as possible, then swallow with a sip or two of water. Also, to settle the stomach take wild, raw honey, either the local type or wild oregano honey, the latter being a digestive aid, two tablespoons three or more times daily. The essence or juice of wild oregano may also prove effective, two tablespoonfuls twice daily. So are the spices fennel and ginger, which always aid in the reduction of nausea. Avoid all solid food until the nausea and vomiting clear. Sip on clear broth soup free of GMOs and MSG. Consume also the wild, raw greens drops, 2 squirts daily. If diarrhea is associated, increase the consumption of both the hemp-wild oregano complex and also the raw honey.

Adrenal exhaustion

In this condition the adrenal glands fail to produce sufficient hormones for optimal health. Stress is a major cause of the syndrome, as is dietary corruption, notably the excessive intake of refined sugar.

Refined sugar causes great corruption in this organ. If it is consumed continously, the adrenal glands can be severely damaged: virtually to the point of no return. The damage can include swelling and internal bleeding within the adrenals. Ultimately, this may result in infection. The most common agent which infects the adrenal glands is tuberculosis. Upon autopsy as many as one-third of Americans have been found to suffer active tuberculosis infection within the part of the gland known as the adrenal cortex.

A crude, unprocessed extract of hemp is an ideal aid for adrenal gland regeneration. This is largely a result of the actions of the hemp on the nerve centers.

Treatment protocol

To treat this condition take the hemp-wild oregano oil combination, five or more drops twice daily. Also, consume the juice of wild oregano, an ounce or more daily and the wild oregano whole food plus *Rhus coriaria* complex, two capsules twice daily. Take also a royal jelly plus adrenal-supporting herbs complex, such as Royal Power, two capsules twice daily. Plus, real plant source Purely C, 2 capsules twice daily, is important for adrenal support. Increase the consumption of sea salt, as this greatly supports adrenal function. Avoid the consumption of refined sugar and excess chocolate, which devastate these glands.

Asthma

One of the most stubborn, persistent of all respiratory conditions there is no medical cure for asthma. Yet, there are a number of natural substances which can help purge this disease from the body. CO_2 hemp extract is one such natural complex.

No doubt, there are imbalances in the nervous innervation in asthma, especially with chronic cases. This is where cannabinoids can be of invaluable use. The disturbed nerve function leads to a condition known as bronchospasm and, thus, the inability to breathe normally. Cannabinoids are bronchodilators and in some studies appear to work as well as common drugs for this purpose.

The bronchodilatation effect appears to be related to normal physiology, in this case of the endocannabinoid system. An agent of that system the cannabinoid anadamide, has a direct action on the bronchial system by easing constriction, that is causing the bronchial tube muscles to relax.

There was yet another benefit from cannabinoid regulation. This internal cannabinoid caused a strong coughing reflex, which can be invaluable in the bringing up of mucous or other irritants. A strong coughing reflex can prove lifesaving in the event of a deep-seated bronchial or lung infection.

Marijuana smoke has been long known to exert this effect. In a study conducted in 1975 published in the *American Journal of Respiratory and Critical Care Medicine* the investigators determined that marijuana smoke caused "an immediate reversal of exercise-induced asthma..." In three human subjects it was found that in a 1976 study the drug reversed experimentally induced bronchospasm in three asthmatic subjects, working nearly as well as a common anti-bronchospasm drug. In summary of this research according to Daniele Piomelli, professor at the University of California Irvine, "marijuana cannabinoids can control coughs in a number of conditions..." through "targeting cannabinoid receptors in the upper airways..." Even so, it must be kept in mind that it is still smoke and that

184 The Cannabis Cure

this is merely a drug-like effect. The smoke itself, loaded with carcinogens, is noxious for asthmatics. For those suffering with respiratory disease any such source of smoke, whether herbal or tobacco—or from wood—should be avoided. Yet, why are the nerves so irritated? This is largely because of inflammation. The inflammation itself is a result of insults, these being due to a variety of causes, including toxic chemical exposure, allergy, and, most importantly, infection.

In fact, mold and fungus infection is a major provocateur of asthma. Asthmatics know very well that their symptoms are often worsened on damp days with high mold counts or that they suffer an aggravation when exposed to mold-tainted indoor air. The mold spores gain entrance to the bronchial and lung tissue, where they aggressively invade. This leads to irritation, making the bronchial tract hypersensitive to stimuli, including airborne mold, dust, pollen, and dander. Regarding allergy, it is largely food intolerance that is the aggravating factor. Key foods which can provoke asthma attacks include corn, wheat, rye, milk products, citrus, and soy. There are chemicals, too, which are provocateurs, including food dyes, artificial flavors, aspartame, brominated vegetable oils, and MSG. Too, in this condition the intake of heavily processed foods must be curtailed, including refined sugar, white flour, refined vegetable oils, and white rice.

Treatment protocol

There are profound benefits in asthma with the intake of CO_2 extract of hemp. Yet, even more sophisticated is the use of wild oregano extracts, both the oil of wild oregano and the raw CO_2 extract. Wild oregano oil has great antiseptic powers against fungi and can be taken as drops under the tongue or in juice/water. It can also be taken as gelcaps. It's a powerful germicide against the main cause of this condition, which is mold as well as candida yeast. To treat this condition take the hemp-wild oregano oil complex, 10 drops two or three times daily. Also take the oil of wild oregano, 10 drops twice daily (they can be taken at the same time). Additionally, for supporting immune health take a whole food, camu camu-based vitamin C complex also containing acerola cherry and the antiseptic *Rhus coriaria*, one or more capsules twice daily. Consume the wild nettle-based greens flushing agent, 40 drops under the tongue twice daily. For tough cases it may be necessary to also consume the multiple spice complex consisting of dessicated oils of wild oregano and sage plus cumin and cinnamon oils: two or more capsules twice daily.

Gastritis and ulcers

There can be no doubt about it high-Beta-caryophyllene herbal medicines are highly protective for stomach and esophageal health. In fact, such herbal complexes are protective for the health of the entire gut. Beta-caryophyllene is the active ingredient of a variety of spices which have well-established roles in supporting stomach and intestinal health. Essentially, the substance can be regarded as a calming agent for both gastric and intestinal function. Moreover, with gastritis and reflux this is sorely needed.

Treatment protocol

The stomach, esophagus, and upper small intestine are highly receptive to cannabinoid therapy. This is largely a function of the action of these compounds on receptor sites, one similar to that of acid-suppressing drugs. Yet, it is also related to direct actions of the cannabinoids and, particularly, Beta-caryophyllene on the gut mucous membranes. For gastric distress of any kind take the hemp-wild oregano complex as sublingual drops, 5 or more drops twice daily. For tough conditions use the super-strength variety, 10 drops twice daily. Also, take the whole crude wild oregano-rhus capsules, two capsules or more twice daily.

Lyme disease

This condition is one of the most valuable arenas for the use of cannabinoid therapy. In this disease the entire nervous system is short-circuited as a result of the tick-borne infestation. The Lyme spirochete is treacherous and readily invades the nervous system. There, it can cause chronic infection, placing great stress on the endocannabinoid system. It may also infect the spinal cord and peripheral nerves. All this leads to great pain and inflammation causing a wide range of symptoms, including head pain, a sensation of disconnect on where the head is versus the rest of the body, mental fog, dizziness, neck stiffness, fullness or stiffness of the spine, tremors, and paralysis. All such symptoms respond to hemp-wild oregano therapy.

Other arenas of invasion include the skin, muscles, joints, bloodstream, and internal organs. This is a powerful germ. The immune system on its own fails to stem the invasion. It must be obliterated through external powers which motivate the immune system into action. This is why cannabinoid-rich hemp and wild oregano extracts are so invaluable. In this regard it must be realized that one of the key destinations of the cannabinoids is the white blood cells themselves. Plus, wild oregano is a germicide and directly attacks and destroys the Lyme spirochete. Beta-caryophyllene is a key mediator against the symptoms and corruptions of Lyme. It is a major discovery. It is substances which are rich in this highly antiinflammatory compound, like wild oregano, rosemary, and sage, along with CO_2 extract of hemp, that are the answer for the cure of this disease. Other key sources of this compound include basil, black pepper, turmeric, parsley, hops, and their extracts.

Treatment protocol

Lyme is one of the most dangerous and stubborn of all chronic diseases known. Usually, it take a considerable effort with large doses to purge it. Take the hemp-wild oregano complex, 10 drops three times daily, using the super-strength for tough cases, 20 drops three times daily. Also, take the super-strength oil of wild oregano, 20 or more drops three times daily; they can be taken at the same time. Consume the multiple spice dessicated oil complex, two or more capsules twice daily. Also, take the whole crude wild oregano-rhus formula, three capsules three times daily. For topical treatment use the bone-activating rubbing oil, rubbing it vigorously over any involved area or joint as often as needed. For more detailed information see the *Lyme Disease Cure* (Knowledge House Publishers, same author).

Cancer

Since the times of ancient Egypt hemp has played a role in cancer treatment. Regardless, it was well known in antiquity that the use of cannabis, medicinally, proved effective in the reversal of chronic disease. With cancer powerful hemp extracts have particularly novel properties. This is true of CBD, so-called CBD oil, the raw whole food leaf/stalk extract, and the organically raised seed oil. In modern science there is a plethora of evidence demonstrating the curative powers of hemp extracts in the treatment of cancer. In particular, colon, breast, and brain cancer have been found to respond positively to cannabinoid therapy.

The beneficial effects are largely related to the regulatory role of these compounds. If there is a corruption in the tissues, the cannabinoids seek it and initiate actions against it. It is these substances which act on the receptor sites, not only for healthy cells but also for the diseased, that is cancerous, ones. Effectively, cannabinoids reprogram the cells, the healthy ones to become healthier and stronger—more resistant to cancer—and also the cancerous ones, in this case to self-destruct, known as apoptosis. It is a rather incredible mechanism achieved by the cannabinoids, that they can reverse the trend and program the cancer cells to essentially kill themselves. This is true not only of cannabidiol but also Beta-caryophyllene, which is one of the most potent inducers of programmed cell death known.

Endocannabinoid receptor blockage in mice leads to negative consequences. In a telling finding it increases the propensity for tumor development, while also causing depression.

Breast tissue does not natively have a major supply of the receptors for circulating endocannabinoids, however, this changes when mutations occur in this organ. When cancer cells develop, that's when the endocannabinoids begin to be found in these tissues. This is a most crucial issue. It demonstrates the immense role played by these compounds and their receptors in regulation. At this point these substances aid in causing programed cell death, while also blocking metastatic formation. The antitumor properties of cannabis are greatly enhanced, in fact, vastly so by the addition of CO_2-extracted wild oregano oil. This is a serious disease and, thus, the highest potency and efficacy is needed. For optimal results be sure that the CO_2 oregano extract is wild and 100% true oregano species, not marjoram, thymus species, GMO, and/or farm-raised. There is a major difference in efficacy. The majority of CO_2-extracted oregano oil available is from marjoram species and/or commercial, farm-raised oregano. As well, the hemp extract must be of the highest quality, preferably organic. It must be extracted only with harmless carbon dioxide, never with alcohol, butane, hexane, or other solvents, the residues of which themselves are carcinogenic.

The issue of residues is a crucial one. Players in the industry will claim their products as solvent-free, saying that there are "no detectable levels." What this means is that, in fact, solvents were used, including the highly carcinogenic hexane, but that the amounts were driven off with heat. There still are residues, but they are purportedly below the 'acceptable' levels. Yet, no one considers; just what do such harsh chemicals do to the delicate molecules of hemp and other plants? Moreover, in particular, harsh chemical solvents are carcinogens and should not be consumed by cancer patients.

Whole food, solvent-free CO_2 extract of wild oregano is far more aggressive as a natural medicinal complex than the farm-raised. Moreover, in some cases farm-raised material is corrupted genetically through genetic engineering. Some one-third of the oregano oil supplements on the market are

GMO-tainted. As mentioned previously wild oregano is a dense source of the all-important compound, Beta-caryophyllene. This gives great power to the wild oregano as an antitumor agent. Yet, it is also the key active ingredient of cold-extracted hemp. In its overall powers Beta-caryophyllene is a more aggressive, effective antitumor agent than cannabidiol alone. In other words, it works more quickly, and universally, in attacking and reversing this disease than cannabidiol or hemp CO_2 extract alone.

Treatment protocol

Regarding cancer, the cannabinoids are one of many classes of natural compounds which are essential to its treatment. Others sources of antitumor complexes include wild berries and their extracts, wild greens and their extracts, organic carrot juice, wild rosemary and its extracts, and far more. To treat this condition take the hemp-wild oregano complex, 20 or more drops three times daily. Also consume the juice of wild oregano, an ounce or more twice daily. Eat as many organic berries as possible and also wild berries, if available. Additionally, consume wild, raw berry extracts, like the super-charged five berries extract, an ounce twice daily. Consume the wild rosemary extract as an aromatic essence, an ounce twice daily. Topically, apply the oil of wild oregano super-strength and also the super-strength form of the hemp-wild oregano extract (beware; it can stain clothes or sheets). Avoid all solvent-extracted forms of cannabis extracts.

Chemotherapy and radiation damage

No doubt, the damage caused to the human body by

chemotherapy and radiotherapy is vast. For instance, many of the commonly used, synthetic chemotherapeutic agents cause wholesale cell destruction, even of brain and nerve cells. Who would want to consume or be infused with a substance that destroys living, vital human cells? Regarding radiation, it is a shot-gun approach at best, destroying, systematically, healthy tissue as well as the diseased type. With natural chemotherapy there is no such destruction. The only cells which are destroyed are the noxious, the toxic, and the disease-causing. The cannabinoids of hemp are natural chemotherapeutic agents. They operate not by directly destroying the diseased cells but, rather, through a more novel, in fact, highly sophisticated mechanism. This is through apoptosis or programmed cell death, where the natural agent induces the self-destruction of cancerous tissue. This is also true of other diseased cells such as those of atheromatous plaques and the sick, corrupt cells of eczema and psoriasis. Natural complexes which fight and reverse the damage induced by chemotherapy and radiation include wild, raw berries extract, wild, raw greens extracts, wild, raw chaga extract, extracts of wild rosemary, oregano, and sage as well as, of course, high-Beta-caryophyllene, CO_2 extract of organic hemp.

Treatment protocol

For persons suffering from chemotherapy-related damage and radiological damage the use of spice extracts should be aggressive, along with the intake of CO_2-extracted hemp. Take 10 to 20 drops of the hemp-wild oregano complex two or three times daily. Additionally, use the oil of wild oregano formula in extra virgin olive oil, five or more drops twice daily, also using this topically, especially on radiation-damaged skin. Consume the juice of wild oregano, an ounce twice daily. As a potent antioxidant to protect the tissues from chemical and radiation damage consume wild turmeric extract, 20 to 40 drops twice daily. Take also wild, raw chaga as sublingual drops, four dropperfuls two or more times daily. For radiation burns use the hemp-wild oregano extract drops, the super-strength wild oregano oil, and/or the hemp-wild oregano cream with wild nettles extract. Chaga cream in a beeswax base can also be used to reverse chemically-induced or radiation-induced skin or tissue damage. Use also the highly effective wild oregano-hemp-wild nettle cream in a base of raw honey and bee propolis, applying as often as needed. Such a cream is a potent natural therapy for all radiation and chemotherapy injuries, especially to the skin, muscles, and nerves.

Chapter Eleven

A Cure for Addictions?

There is much need for a simple, easy-to-administer cure for addiction syndromes. Now, it is well established that people are readily addicted to drugs. This is true not only for illicit ones but also the prescription types, which is, ultimately, the most common type of drug addiction. Drugs which are habit forming include heroin, cocaine, crack, ecstasy, codeine, marijuana, and amphetamines. Prescription drugs which are highly addictive include sleeping medications and mood-altering agents, the so-called SSRIs such as Valium, Xanax, Paxil, Effexor, and others. Of course, all opiates are addictive, and many addictions occur as a consequence of medical treatment. Yet, far more common than drug dependency is addiction to alcohol. So, let us begin with this, the most poisonous, destructive, and deadly of all drugs.

194 The Cannabis Cure

Alcoholism

Beer, wine, and hard liquor, in particular, can all be addicting. Globally, there are hundreds of millions of alcoholics. All such individuals are suffering great destructive effects on their bodies. Then, too, usually, they cause damage and destruction to others, including their loved ones and, in fact, any of those who are close to them. At all costs alcoholism must be cured. All it causes is devastation, for the individual, for loved ones, for friends, and for the entire society at-large.

For alcoholics the goal is to alter the nerve centers, essentially, to deaden them. Physiologically, this is precisely what it does. They are self-treating their bodies with a poison to manipulate mood sensations. With rare exceptions by no means are people drinking alcohol merely as a culinary experience. In most cases alcoholic beverages have a horrid taste, even many wines. The substance itself is a toxin produced by bacteria, the purpose of which is to destroy its enemies. Therefore, it is a poisonous substance, make no mistake about it. Regardless, who feels refreshed and enlivened after consuming such beverages? Instead people lose their senses and often become agitated, in some cases violent.

In the brain the endocannabinoid system acts to regulate key organ systems, in fact, virtually all such systems from the thinking parts to those which automatically regulate body functions. Alcohol disrupts this regulatory role. In fact, the substance categorically destroys both the internally produced cannabinoids and their receptor sites, while also destroying the cells that act upon the neurons.

The motor and thinking centers of the brain are cannabinoid-dependent. Then, what are the primary symptoms of chronic alcohol intoxication? These symptoms include memory loss, agitation, fits of rage, decrease in motor or muscular capacity, muscle atrophy, paresthesias, reduced body core temperature, and catalepsy, that is loss of sensation in the body characterized by a trance-like state, essentially a seizure.

Are these, then, a sign of alcohol-induced chemical imbalances? It would seem to be the case, since all such symptoms and corruptions are associated with endocannabinoid deficiency and, certainly, with the diminution of the normal transmission of nerve impulses. Moreover, they are all reversed through the intake of goodly doses of dietary cannabinoids.

In fact, alcohol irritates or, shall it be said, excites the endocannabinoid receptors. Rapidly, these receptors develop a dependency on this substance. This is why the cannabinoids are so invaluable for the treatment of this disease. They act to replace the irritational effects of alcohol and, thus, aid in the reversal of the addiction. Essentially, they block the noxious actions of alcohol on these protein-based receptors.

In experimental models chronic alcohol consumption was found to have a measurable effect on the internally produced cannabinoids, causing them to be concentrated in nerve cells. This is a defense mechanism, an attempt to preserve these signaling agents or at least an attempt by the neurons at self-protection. In this regard it should be kept in mind that alcohol is a deliberate nerve cell poison. A mere single high-ball is capable of destroying some one million brain cells. What could be more poisonous than this? Yet, ultimately, with continued consumption the levels of the endocannabinoids decrease, and rapidly, there is a decline in the levels of these crucial compounds within the center of the brain, known as the mid-brain. In any case, clearly, alcohol has a disruptive effect on the internal cannabinoid system, eventually causing not only a reduction in the levels of these substances but also the destruction and loss of the receptor sites themselves. In fact, cannabinoids activate the same sensation pathways, often called reward pathways, as does alcohol. Yet, the latter damages the receptor sites, while the former preserves them. Too, cannabinoids aid in the control of food intake, while through its destructive effects on brain tissue alcoholic beverages suppress it.

Even so, nothing could be more harmful to the human body than hard liquor. Systematically, this substance corrupts human organs and cells. It is exceedingly toxic to the brain, obliterating nerve cells by the tens of millions with every bottle consumed. It is also highly toxic to the liver and stomach, where it kills millions of cells per dose.

Here is a key issue. Initially, alcohol causes a rise in mood-controlling substances, like endorphins and cannabinoids. It also increases the tone of cannabinoid receptors. The rise or benefit, the reward, is short-lived.

An increase in tone means the receptors are more vigorous in receiving these compounds. This is crucial, since it explains the temporary high or let it be said mood reaction gained by the consumption of this substance. Regarding endorphins, the types induced by alcohol are addictive substances released from the front of the brain. This in part explains why people claim they 'feel good' or 'better' after drinking.

The study, performed by J. Mitchell of the University of California San Francisco, determined that for certain people alcohol causes "endorphins to be released" in the frontal cortex. Both heavy drinkers and non-drinkers were given alcohol after which endorphin levels and any sensations were assessed. Not surprisingly, the volunteers who drank the booze reported enjoyable "feelings of pleasure." It was also discovered that the alcoholics reacted in yet another way, becoming intoxicated at the higher endorphin levels, which did not occur in the non-drinkers. This gives a clue for the degree of the addiction; alcoholics drink just so they can become wasted, mentally, into oblivion.

By creating an internal sense of calm, peace, and, perhaps, happiness cannabinoids would replace this. That is why they are ideal for the treatment of this disease. Essentially, cannabinoids—CBD and its fellow compounds—are the body's means of protection against alcohol toxicity. Here is a curious result in humans. In a study conducted by P. Consroe published in *Psychopharmacology* humans were given alcohol or the drug, along with CBD oil. In those given the combination blood levels were lower than in those who just received alcohol. This indicates that cannabinoids have a direct action in the purging or detoxification of this substance.

The cannabinoids also directly protect the brain from alcohol-induced toxicity. According to US investigators at the NIH in testing of binge alcohol exposure CBD oil had a marked effect in protecting neuronal tissue from toxicity. The greater the dose the higher was the degree of protection. The conclusion by investigators was that cannabinoid-rich supplements blocked the degenerative actions of alcohol on brain tissue, including the expected degeneration of the cerebral cortex. This makes sense, since much of this damage is mediated by free radicals, and herbal medicines, such as hemp, are antioxidants, blocking such damage.

Binge alcohol drinking always causes a degree of damage to nerve tissue, especially the higher brain. The study provided definitive evidence that hemp extracts prevent such damage, so at a minimum they must be taken in the immediate aftermath. The results were enhanced through the addition of fat soluble antioxidants, notably vitamin E, proving the role of free radical-induced lipid oxidation as a result of alcohol ingestion.

This is why the addition of antioxidant-rich, flavonoid-dense wild oregano extract is so crucial to cannabinoid therapy. The fact is second only to clove extract wild oregano oil is the most potent antioxidant known. No synthetic antioxidant, such as BHT, alpha tocopherol, or beta carotene, can match its powers. Additionally, the wild oregano antioxidants, which include vitamin E and beta carotene, along with potent phenolic compounds, like carvacrol and Beta-caryophyllene, help maintain the molecular powers of cannabis extract, preventing their oxidation while also increasing their absorption.

This substance, in particular, Beta-caryophyllene is effective versus addictions even more so than all the other cannabinoids combined. German investigators discovered that this substance vigorously binds to the marijuana pathways in the body. Specifically, it binds to the CB2 receptors. This is why it is a potent anti-anxiety and antidepressive agent. In this regard according to a report in *Trends in Pharmacological Sciences*, "epidemiological studies have indicated that the most common self-reported reason for using cannabis is rooted in its ability to reduce feelings of stress, tension, and anxiety." This is why it is ideal for the treatment of addiction syndromes.

Treatment protocol

A hemp-wild oregano complex as sublingual drops or gelcaps is an ideal treatment for alcohol addiction. This is a result of actions by the hemp-oregano cannabinoids, which mimic those of alcohol. It is also a consequence of the powerful actions of these two herbal extracts in halting oxidative damage in the brain. Consider the hemp-wild oregano combination an antidote to alcohol addiction. To treat this disease take 10 or more drops of this complex as often as necessary. At every severe craving for alcohol it should be consumed. For extreme cases use the super-strength form, 10 to 20 drops as often as needed. This will create a great sense of calm and reduce the addictive desire for this drug. This therapy may be supported through the intake of a hemp-sprouted brown rice protein powder, two tablespoonful sin juice, water, or almond milk twice daily. Additionally, take a whole food, non-GMO vitamin E source, such as Purely-E drops, 10 drops twice daily. Additionally, consume a whole food B complex powder, 2 T. daily.

Drug addiction in general

No doubt, raw cannabis extract is one of the most potent therapeutic agents for the reversal of drug addiction. Raw extract of wild oregano is also no minor player, being an antidote to chemical and drug toxicity. In one study cocaine toxicity was addressed through the intake of cannabinoids. Published in *Mediators of Inflammation,* here, a rat study was performed where the animals were intoxicated with cocaine, developing significant seizures and liver toxicity. The administration of CBD oil protected against this toxicity, abolishing the cocaine-induced seizures. A high dose of CBD oil, some 30 mg per kilogram, reduced the acute liver toxicity. This proved that to protect the liver from chemical toxicity the ingestion of cannabinoid-rich foods and/or supplements is essential.

In drug addiction there are great imbalances in neurotransmission. This is in part the reason for the dependency. People get a temporary reaction, a high or a lift, from the drugs. So, they go to them repeatedly. If there were sufficient levels of naturally occurring or outside-source neurotransmitters, then, the dependency upon drugs would be eliminated.

Two key neurotransmitters which are deficient and/or dysfunctional in drug addiction, are GABA and dopamine. Cannabinoids increase the activity of both these neurotransmitters. Notes Baye in *New Research on Alcoholism* cannabinoids increase the release of dopamine within brain tissue, which is precisely the goal of many drugs for the treatment of addiction.

Now, it should be kept in mind that this is the way to get high with illicit drugs, as well as the prescription kind: this temporary rise in the neurotransmitter load. Here, cannabinoids achieve a miracle. While they are capable of improving the production and release of key neurotransmitters, such as GABA, dopamine, and serotonin, see what they do after the administration of drugs, like alcohol. They halt the ability in test models of acute alcohol consumption to cause an artificial rise in dopamine. Moreover, while cannabinoids improve the capacity of nerve cells to send key impulsions, drugs depress and corrupt them. Thus, once again, the role of the cannabinoids is to normalize nerve function, whether it is excessively depressed or excitable.

It's a signaling system, after all. How can putting the body on notice for key signals be anything other than normalization? In contrast, noxious synthetic or refined drugs, like cocaine, heroin, codeine, and alcohol, contribute nothing to the native signaling mechanisms. Rather, these agents thoroughly corrupt them, pharmaceutical drugs being the most notorious in this regard. It is a curious issue that the federal government places so much emphasis on marijuana. Simultaneously, nothing is done to deal with the more highly fatal drugs: alcohol and tobacco as well as pharmaceutical agents. In fact, the purpose of the federal system is to largely protect these monopolies. Consider vaccines, which cause hundreds of fatalities in Americans yearly. These are sudden fatalities, which occur within a few hours or days after the injections. The greatest victims are infants and children, innocents, who are essentially murdered by these septic solutions. Yet, nothing is done about it. Instead, the federal government endorses it, immunizing, no pun intended, the drug companies from prosecution. If marijuana is to be banned, then, surely inoculations, SSRIs, acetaminophen, and other death-producers must also be similarly banned. This will never happen. Thus, it is pure hypocrisy, make no mistake about it.

Tobacco addiction

Tobacco smoking is one of the most obnoxious, destructive, and dangerous of all addictive habits. At all costs the habit must be eliminated, as it causes great corruption, both to the smoking individual and all who are around such a one. Tobacco is a major cause of fatality, largely through an increased incidence of heart disease and cancer. It also causes fatality through direct damage to the lungs. The often fatal conditions COPD and emphysema are the result of gradual, systematic tobacco-smoke induced lung destruction. As a smoking agent tobacco is far more toxic than marijuana. Regardless, it is the premise, here, that no plant matter should be regularly and routinely smoked as a result of the damage this causes to human tissues.

Treatment protocol

To treat this condition take the hemp-wild oregano complex as sublingual drops, 10 drops under the tongue two or more times; or take a few drops with every craving for cigarettes. Also, take the oil of wild oregano as sublingual drops, three to five drops several times daily. For adrenal support take a high-quality royal jelly supplement, two capsules three times daily. Never give up. It is possible to quit: without nicotine-based drugs.

Pot addiction

Is it possible that a form of marijuana, industrial cannabis, can be used to treat high-THC pot addiction? In fact, this is precisely the case, since the primary active ingredients of the industrial type, the CB2 receptor activating cannabinoids, directly antagonize the actions of THC.

Make no mistake about it high-THC pot is highly addictive. The degree of the addiction varies in individuals, with those with weak adrenals being the most vulnerable to difficulty in withdrawing. Moreover, chronic regular smokers in particular have difficulty achieving a symptom-free, smooth withdrawal. That transition is greatly facilitated through the intake of non-psychoactive hemp, especially the type combined with wild oregano.

Treatment protocol

To treat this condition take the hemp-wild oregano complex as sublingual drops, 10 drops under the tongue two or more times daily. Also, in the event of heavy metal overload or chemical toxicity take the total body purging agent, one ounce or more daily for at least one month. Consume also the juice of wild oregano, one ounce or more daily, along with the dessicated spice complex, two capsules twice daily. If swallowing is difficult, use the wild multiple spice drops, 20 drops twice daily. The aromatic essence of wild oregano, wild sage, wild rosemary, plus rose and orange blossom may prove invaluable, an ounce twice daily. The consumption of wild chaga-birch bark tea is advised, 2 to 3 cups daily.

Sugar addiction

What can a person do about sugar addiction? It is simple. All that is needed is to take the same approach as all the other addictions, which is to boost and facilitate the signaling mechanisms. Another key approach is to deal with blood sugar imbalances and also fungal overload. When the blood sugar mechanism is disturbed, obviously, people not only crave sugar but also vigorously consume it. Regarding fungi, this is a major issue in regard to cravings. The fungi secrete chemicals which cause the addict to consume sugar, often in large quantities.

In most cases sugar addicts are anxiety-ridden. In other cases they are chronically depressed. In all instances such addicts suffer internal agitation. Often, this depletes the system so severely that the main symptom becomes extreme fatigue. The person can no longer function, and the high or benefit gained from eating sugar or drinking sugar-infested drinks is temporary at best. Some people can eliminate the addiction cold-turkey. However, for extreme, unrelenting addiction it may be necessary to take the appropriate supplements to facilitate the cure. This includes the vigorous use of oil of wild oregano to purge the fungal and yeast overload, which automatically exists as a result of routine consumption of this noxious substance.

Treatment protocol

To treat this condition take the hemp-wild oregano complex, 5 to 10 drops under the tongue two or more times daily. Also, consume the aromatic essence of wild oregano, wild sage, wild rosemary, plus rose and orange blossom, one ounce twice daily. Aggressively purge the fungus/yeast by taking the oil of wild oregano, 10 drops three times daily. Also, support the pancreatic and liver systems, that is the blood sugar mechanisms, with the specialized spice drops for regulating insulin consisting of oils of cumin, cinnamon, oregano, and fenugreek, five drops under the tongue as often as needed, especially when craving sugar.

Chapter Twelve

Treating Hormonal Imbalances

The body produces the endocrine secretions, the hormones, as agents of control. All such endocrine secretions serve the sole purpose as chemical messengers. The hormones and cannabinoids work as a team to maintain the health-producing controlling mechanisms that keep the body in good order. To maintain optimal function of the key regulatory glands of the hormone system, for instance, the hypothalmus, pineal, pituitary, adrenals, and thyroid, the regular intake of cannabinoids is ideal. In this regard it must be remembered that the hormone system is under nervous control. If that nervous system is in disarray, the endocrine glands will correspondingly be under duress, and this may lead to a variety of symptoms of imbalances, which may be directly related to a deficit in cannabinoids.

So, then, there can be a deficiency of both hormonal secretions, like thyroid hormone, adrenal hormones, testosterone, and estrogen, as well as the endocannabinoids themselves. There may also simply be a deficiency in the intake of dietary cannabinoids. Regardless, in all cases of dysfunctional and/or stressed hormonal glands, the wild oregano-hemp complex is invaluable. In contrast, psychoactive hemp, actually, marijuana is destructive to the hormone glands. These glands are readily disturbed by the slightest degree of toxicity and corruption. As mentioned previously the intake, for instance, of any kind of smoke, whether from cigarettes, marijuana, or mere wood, disturbs them.

The pineal and pituitary

It is the cannabinoids which exert profound actions in the signaling of nerve impulses. Thus, one of the greatest domains of their actions is within the brain tissue itself. Housed within that tissue are key endocrine glands, including the so-called ultimate master glands, the pituitary and the pineal. Both these glands are readily disturbed by nervous stress. They are also highly vulnerable to oxidative damage. That is why the regular antioxidant-rich hemp-wild oregano formula is ideal. Furthermore, for balance to be achieved the signaling mechanisms need to be re-established. To do so requires an increase in the synthesis of the internal cannabinoid as well as an increase in dietary or supplemental consumption of dietary ones. No wonder people get a feel-good response from the intake of cinnamon, cloves, oregano, thyme, rosemary, parsley, sage, and black pepper.

Treatment protocol

To boost the function of these glands take the hemp-wild oregano formula, five to 10 drops under the tongue twice daily.

Also, take the neurologically activating aromatic essence complex consisting of essences of rosemary, sage, oregano, rose petal, and orange blossom, a half ounce or more daily. For extreme cases of dysfunction also take the juice of wild oregano, a half ounce once or twice daily.

Thyroid function

Because of its dependence on regulatory systems the thyroid gland greatly benefits from hemp extract therapy. Wild oregano is also a highly beneficial agent for supporting thyroid health. While it surprises people the thyroid gland can readily become infected by a number of pathogens, including viruses, bacteria, fungi, and parasites. Additionally, it is highly vulnerable to radiation-induced damage. A hemp-wild oregano complex is, therefore, ideal for supporting the health of this organ.

Treatment protocol

Regarding the thyroid the importance of the cannabinoids is in regulation of hormone production and secretion. To support the health of this gland take the hemp-wild oregano combination, five drops under the tongue twice daily. For severe conditions, including significant inflammation in the organ, as in Grave's or Hashimoto's disease, increase the dose to 10 drops twice daily. It may also be rubbed topically on the thyroid region, as can the oil of wild oregano.

Adrenal function

There is no organ system in the body more vulnerable to the toxicity of mental stress than the adrenal glands. Nervous agitation is highly destructive to these glands. Fear, anxiety, and anger all corrupt it. Controlling or minimizing these emotions, then, aids the function of this gland by decreasing the stress upon it. Regardless, any degree of nervous agitation depletes these glands. That's why the regular intake of cannabinoid-rich spices and spice extracts is so crucial. Furthermore, the fluctuations in blood sugar deplete these glands, as they must make glucocorticoids to help balance blood sugar levels. Caryophyllene-rich spices and foods, notably cinnamon, cloves, wild oregano, cumin, and CO_2 hemp extract, help normalize blood sugar levels.

Treatment protocol

To maintain optimal adrenal function take the hemp-wild oregano complex, five or more drops under the tongue twice daily. Also, take the juice of wild oregano, a half ounce once or twice daily, along with whole food vitamin C from camu camu and acerola cherry, one capsule twice daily. Additionally, increase the consumption of Beta-caryophyllene-rich spices, including cinnamon, clove, cumin, black pepper, oregano, rosemary, and sage.

Can marijuana cause impotence?

Make no mistake about it high-THC marijuana has significant, negative effects on the sexual and fertility apparatus. THC itself directly inhibits the secretion of key pituitary hormones, including LH, FSH, and prolactin. It is simply too strong for the endocrine organs of the brain, which it readily overloads. All such hormones are crucial for fertility and lactation. Studies on primates demonstrate that marijuana-induced disruption of these hormone systems leads to disruption of ovulation and sperm production. It is thought that this toxicity is a consequence of THC's actions on the actions of the hypothalmus. The proof of this toxicity appears to be undeniable. In animal models chronic exposure leads to a drop in not only LH and FSH but also testosterone. This leads to dysfunction in the prostate, seminal vesicles, and testes. Marijuana raises the levels in the body of a key pro-inflammatory compound, prostaglandin E-2. This leads to a wide range of undesired consequences, including inflammation in the arteries and brain as well as a constriction in blood flow to this organ. Ultimately, this may negatively effect the control centers for hormone synthesis, leading to a progressive drop in testosterone synthesis. The same is seen in humans who chronically ingest the smoke.

A number of the chemicals in marijuana smoke are poisonous to brain cells. This can lead to a deadening of the nerves, causing a drop in the production of key neurotransmitters within the brain, including acetylcholine. Precursors needed to cause dilation of the blood vessels, such as nitric oxide, become depressed, although in some cases the levels become dramatically elevated before such depression occurs. The nervous system's capacity for proper sexual function and for the creation of healthy erections becomes exhausted. As a result, it becomes difficult to have an erection let alone maintain one.

Because of the constant exposure to the drug the nerve cell capacity becomes corrupted. The brain and its connections operate in confusion, with poor capacity of interconnection. Orgasm may now fail or become feeble. Sperm and seminal fluid is in decline. Chromosomal aberrations occur. There is ultimately a full depletion of

210 The Cannabis Cure

messenger hormones. The gonads, therefore, begin to atrophy: to shrink. Ultimately, the chronic marijuana user becomes impotent. This is true of any smoker, whether of pot or tobacco; however, because of its toxic effects on the hormonal signaling mechanism marijuana is particularly noxious in this regard.

Treatment protocol

In the treatment of marijuana-induced impotence it is crucial to take one strong action, which is to avoid the consumption of high-THC marijuana in any form. Take as an antidote the wild oregano-hemp CO_2-extracted complex, five to 10 drops once or twice daily. To strengthen the sexual apparatus consume royal jelly, two or more capsules daily. To create balance in the neuro-endocrine system take the aromatic essence of rose water, orange blossom, sage, oregano, and rosemary, an ounce once or twice daily. Be sure to increase the consumption of healthy animal fat from free-range eggs, grass-fed milk products, and grass-fed meat, all of which are rich in testosterone-like hormones.

Bone disease

Is bone disease a hormonal disorder? To a large degree the hormones control bone health. Consider the substances which have the greatest power over the skeleton: vitamin D, testosterone, estrogen, parathyroid hormone, calcitonin, and thyroid hormone. All are endocrine secretions.

There is a wide range of illnesses which can afflict the skeletal system. In addition to hormonal deficiency the skeleton may break down as a result of nutritional deficiency. It may even be attacked by germs. Both chronic and acute infections may occur. Serious infection of bone tissue is known as osteomyelitis. Furthermore, whether from injury or infection inflammation readily develops in the bones, leading to pain and disability. Diseases of the bone include osteoporosis, Paget's disease, Pott's disease (due to TB infection), spinal stenosis, and bone cancer. In addition, bones can be attacked as a result of distant cancers, where the malignant tissue is seeded to the skeleton, attacking it. This is known as metastatic bone disease. It all represents a loss of tissue control systems, where the disease processes are wreaking havoc upon the boney skeleton.

Regarding skeletal and bone health hemp extracts and/or hemp foods are highly beneficial. When considering the nature of the plant this makes great sense. The fibers of hemp are among the strongest, toughest plant fibers known. Moreover, the true hemp, the industrial type, is one of the straightest-growing, tallest herbal plants in existence. So, if a person wishes to stand tall and strong, even in old age, hemp is essential. Moreover, the bones are a major site of action for the cannabanoids, since they are peppered with CB2 receptors.

Extracts of hemp have direct actions on bone matter. This is true of the cold-pressed seed oil, the seed protein, and the raw, organic, crude whole food CO_2 extract.

The CO_2, whole food extract is one of the most potent bone builders known. One of the key reasons for this is the rich content of that all-important hemp component, Beta-caryophyllene. This compound helps prevent degeneration of the bones by boosting the synthesis of new bone. Simultaneously, it helps halt inflammatory processes within the skeletal system. Both hemp and wild oregano are dense sources of this substance. Moreover, hempseed protein and the seed itself are top sources of magnesium, a mineral needed to enhance bone density. There is another obvious reason for the beneficial action of hemp extracts. This relates to the signaling mechanisms of the body, that regulatory entity known as the endocannabinoid system. Activation of this system is much needed to aid and create a state of powerful health for the bones. It is to reverse inflammation and bone loss. It is also to, thus, induce healing in diseased bone. Plus, the normalization of this signaling can act directly on the diseased tissue, particularly the cancerous matter, causing the cancer cells to die through self-destruction.

Wild oregano extracts achieve the same feat. Once again, it is largely a consequence of the Beta-caryophyllene content, yet it is also a result of the action of the wild oregano phenols, which destroy cancer cells. Other spice oil complexes which build bone health and destroy cancerous tissue include extracts of wild rosemary, sage, thyme, fir, and pine. These aromatic spice oils are among the most powerful bone pain- and inflammation-relieving agents known. In addition, the whole spices themselves are bone-building agents, particularly when combined with raw bone from New Zealand grass-fed cattle.

Treatment protocol

In the treatment of bone disorders it is crucial to use all the various forms of hemp medicines and/or nutritional supplements. Take the hemp-wild oregano high Beta-caryophyllene complex, 10 or more drops twice daily. This oil can also be rubbed over the diseased bone site. For generalized bone disease it can be rubbed or applied to the soles of the feet, which represent the skeleton, and also the long bones: the tibia and top of the femur. Consume also organic hempseed oil, two tablespoonfuls daily. Take a hempseed protein combined, ideally, with wild chaga and sprouted brown rice protein powder, three tablespoonsful daily. Take the bone-activating wild rosemary, wild oregano, and wild sage capsules, along with raw bone from New Zealand grass-fed cattle, two or more capsules twice daily. Use the bone-activating rubbing oil consisting of oils of wild sage, rosemary, and oregano, applied topically on the soles of the feet and rubbed up-and-down the spine, also along the long bones. Additionally, the hormone system must be bolstered. A key, here, is to be sure to get extra doses of vitamin D but not the synthetic type, rather, the entirely natural complex. This is best achieved through the intake of fatty wild salmon oil, a dense source of natural vitamin D plus vitamin A: take three or more capsules twice daily. The top food sources of vitamin D include organic liver, whole milk products, fish roe, and egg yolks. Never give up. The bone tissue can be healed. It just takes aggressive therapy plus persistence.

Chapter Thirteen

Animals and Cannabis

With pets, great caution must be taken regarding marijuana. Even with the medicinal type care must be taken. The drug itself is highly toxic to them where, in particular, its resin can poison pets rapidly. For instance, cats and dogs have no means to metabolize it efficiently. Thus, it readily damages their internal organs, particularly their nervous systems. Pets suffering from marijuana intoxication often show impaired balance. Their heads wobble. They may stagger, stumble, and fall attempting to walk. With acute intoxication vomiting, diarrhea, and drooling may develop. With heavy exposure they often lose bowel and bladder control, which also, by the way, can occur in humans.

The sensory stimuli of these animals is corrupted. They may thus over-react to noises, movements, even touch. This may be manifested by trembling of their bodies and/or jerking reactions that resemble seizures. In fact, seizure-like reactions may result, which is a medical emergency. All this can occur through either the inhalation of the smoke or, in particular, the consumption of the plant matter. The toxicity of marijuana is accentuated by the simultaneous intake of other drugs such as alcohol, refined sugar, and theobromine.

There have been fatalities, too. In investigations in Colorado it was found that the toxicity can be extreme. Pets, in this case mainly dogs, develop depression, which, of course, virtually never occurs in such animals but also tremors, twitching, wobbliness, shaking of the head, and vomiting. Colorado investigators also documented seizures in canines. Ultimately, in some cases the pets fell into comas and died.

In pets the loss of the ability to walk, known as ataxia, is surely a most significant sign and must always be taken seriously. So is listlessness, a common consequence of the intoxication. There is also a significant drop in body temperature, known as hypothermia, a most serious sign, one that often precedes fatality. Additionally, often, the animal's eyes become dilated and it may lose its desire for both food and water.

Th heart-beat can slow, or it can rise up. There may be overall agitation and excessive or abnormal vocalization.

The neurotoxic effects of cannabis ingestion in animals typically occur within a half hour to two hours after ingestion and usually last for about 12 hours. However, they can last for days, because the cannabinoids are stored in fat. The extreme toxicity of marijuana ingestion is demonstrated by the following case history:

CASE HISTORY: I go out to get a beer and come back, dog dead on the floor.

It turns out, he ate my weed brownies. (Expletive deleted) that weed.

Clearly, people take it lightly that it is just "weed," that is "It's just an herb—it's natural; it can't do much harm." It was S. Meola, veterinarian of Wheat Ridge, Colorado, who helped put together the study that revealed the danger. Said Meola in an interview with CBS Channel 4, "I just want dogs, kids to be safe. It needs to be treated like any other drug. If you came home with a prescription of Vicodin from your doctor, you wouldn't just leave it sitting there."

The danger was seconded by J. Schoedler, a veterinarian at Alpine Animal Hospital, who has treated dogs sickened by marijuana for decades. Speaking to the *Durango Herald* she noted, "Dogs love the stuff. I've seen them eat the buds, plants, joints, and marijuana in food." Schoedler added that just as dark chocolate is safe for humans to ingest but potentially poisonous to dogs, that same is true of marijuana for dogs. This clearly demonstrates the danger of keeping hallucinogenic marijuana in access to these pets.

Recently, a dog consumed an entire batch of pot-based brownies purchased by the owner at a medical marijuana dispensary. For the owner and her friends it started out as a humorous matter, but that ended quickly. Noted L. Higgins, an emergency room veterinarian at Aspen Meadow Veterinary Specialists in Longmont, "...by the time the dog came to me, she was nearly comatose, nearly dead."

This dog survived. Yet, consider it. Attracted to the cannabis, the dog devoured the plate of brownies and consumed not only the drug but also loads of refined sugar and chocolate, both of which are toxic to such animals. Who in their right minds would consume hallucinogenic marijuana in a base of sugar and chocolate? These are carnivores. They are not meant to eat such sugar-infested drugs. Moreover, who could possibly feel comfortable keeping these THC laced edibles readily accessible, where they could be dangerously consumed by pets and children? "The problem is a person will have one brownie, but a dog gets up on the counter and eats the whole tray," said Fitzgerald. "Their natural instinct is to gorge."

These were accidental cases of poisoning. Far more wretched is the forceful consumption with vulnerable creatures such as pets and children. The deliberate feeding of marijuana to dogs and other pets is an act of great corruption. So is the purposeful exposure of such animals to intoxicating marijuana smoke.

People feed their dogs beer. They will lap it up vigorously. It is no joke; alcohol is exceedingly toxic to them. So is pot, chocolate, and sugar. Animals are fully vulnerable while under the human domain. No one should knowingly abuse them, especially with consumable items. No pets of any kind should be fed intoxicants. These pets have been put in human trust as a gift from the creator. To abuse them in any way is a crime against the animal kingdom.

How to reverse marijuana poisoning in pets

Seek medical attention immediately. If possible, give the pet a drop or two of oil of wild oregano, an antidote to intoxicant poisoning. Also, squirt the greens flushing agent, orally, two more dropperfuls multiple times. The CO_2 extract of hemp plus CO_2 oregano may prove helpful, by blocking the toxicity of THC: start slowly with one or two drops in the mouth. If it is well-tolerated, repeat the dose. Do not give CBD oil. It may prove too strong in sedation, making the situation worse. Only the whole food, crude extract, that is the wild oregano-hemp combination, should be given in this instance, along with wild oil of oregano therapy.

Chapter Fourteen

The FDA and Hemp

What does the FDA say about hemp? In fact, it says very little. Most of its dictates are regarding CBD oil, which it claims is not a legitimate dietary supplement. At a minimum it holds that regarding the cannabidiols no dietary supplement claims can be made. In other words, incredibly, no one can say on labels just what such supplements can do. Even so, no doubt, marijuana is a drug. This is particularly true in its most commonly used form, which is the dried, flowering plant. Rich in resin, which is a dense source of psychoactive agents, this dried plant matter is smoked. Sometimes, it is eaten. Most people use it for its mood-altering properties, that is they take it to get high. They smoke it, because of its effects on the brain, not for any health-related purposes. Thus, it is under the domain of not the FDA but, rather, the Drug Enforcement Agency or DEA.

It can also be deemed an intoxicant, just like alcohol. Intoxicants may be described as substances which have the propensity for being abused. In this regard they create temporary sensations that may in some instances appear beneficial while upon elimination after prolonged use lead to withdrawal symptoms. Intoxicants are also substances which alter the senses, often in a dramatic way, in some cases causing potentially dangerous hallucinations. Examples of such agents include:

- heroin
- cocaine
- codeine and other opiates
- coca leaf and its extracts
- LSD
- ecstasy
- wine
- beer
- hard liquor
- marijuana and/or hashish

Tobacco is yet another commonly consumed addictive substance. Like marijuana and alcohol it is never consumed for health purposes. In some respects marijuana has food value: vitamins, minerals, and more. Yet, so does to a small degree wine in the form of colorful flavonoids and beer in the form of traces of minerals and B vitamins. However, the point is no one consumes them for this purpose. In fact, alcohol actually causes extensive depletion of nutrients from the body, especially magnesium and the B vitamins. Tobacco is a noxious complex that offers nothing positive for human health, rather, only causing vast harm. In this regard it should be banned from human use. It is purely destructive, far more so than marijuana.

One issue is certain. When consumed on a regular or daily basis, the benefits of alcohol and tobacco are far outweighed by the drawbacks, which include the onset of serious diseases as well as premature death. Tobacco is so toxic that people in near association to the smoker are also harmed. This is to such a degree that the incidence of cancer for these innocent by-standers rises significantly. In fact, mere exposure to second hand smoke can directly induce a wide range of cancers, including lung, prostate, breast, and blood cancers. In excess all addictive substances can prove noxious. Yet, what if the drug is specifically created to be ultra-intoxicating? This is surely the case with 'modern' marijuana. Bred to be addictive, it is banned with good cause. Yet, the platform is skewed. The far more destructive, even more addictive, tobacco and alcohol are given a free pass with their consumption having no criminal punishment: that is for self-use. Even so, no one can doubt that marijuana, too, is highly addictive. None of them are safe for human consumption.

Regarding industrial hemp it is not addictive to any degree. In contrast, with pot as a result of the dense amount of THC the resinous matter is unfit for human consumption. Moreover, make no mistake about it this type of marijuana is a hallucinogen. Then, what is such a substance? It is a compound which "Under its influence people see images, hear sounds, and feel sensations that appear to be real but are not. In some cases the intake of hallucinogens leads to rapid, intense emotional swings," which many people are never prepared for. Who in their right mind would want to consume a hallucinogen?

It's quite bizarre, since in many of cannabis' forms it is completely safe for human use. For instance, in the raw plant, that is the juiced plant matter, there is little to none of this psychoactive chemical found. Nor is it found to any major degree in the cold-pressed seed oil, or, if found, it is only in minor amounts.

Even if pot smoking remains illegal this has nothing to do with either medical marijuana or the use of the non-psychoactive type. Laws are being loosened, it is presumed, for the purpose of making the drug-type available for palliative care. The situation is complex. The loosening of laws has both its pros and cons. Derogatory consequences have included acute psychosis and in some cases death by suicide.

It is a very simple issue, though, to deal with. Moreover, it could be done in a not-so-costly manner at the state level. States could simply ban the growth of high-THC marijuana, while fully legalizing the growth, and use, of all other types. It's drug dealers who produce these intoxicating plants. By no means should this type of marijuana be legalized. What good will that do? How will it help anyone? How will burdening society with yet another addictive, hallucinogenic substance do any good? Regarding alcohol and tobacco, little can be done at the governmental level. They are too deeply embedded within Western civilization. The only option is extensive education: to warn people of the great dangers they pose to society and people individually.

The so-called drug wars are yet another issue. That is just as dangerous as free use of marijuana, if not more so. How in the world can people get such extensive prison terms for mere possession, for instance, of this drug? No one gets prison time for alcohol possession, and this is even more dangerous than pot, causing a greater amount of death, destruction, and despair than all other commonly consumed intoxicants combined.

The federal government's blockade of industrial hemp is a dilemma. Freeing up these laws would be invaluable, since, as a result, there would be a non-intoxicating "medical cannabis" available for all who desire it. Moreover, when taken therapeutically it is more effective and more lasting than marijuana smoke could ever be.

Getting the priorities straight: bringing back industrial hemp

A sound approach is to fully legalize industrial marijuana, that is extracts of the standard, food-grade hemp plant. All states should break down existing laws which ban its growth and production. The FDA itself considers certain parts of hemp notably the seeds and its oil or protein to be food-based products. As such, from its perspective there are no legal restrictions against it. Even so, the growth of the actual plant is still largely banned. Here, in the most industrialized country in existence the growth of the world's most versatile, useful crop is effectively prohibited, only allowed for research purposes. It is ludicrous. This is also highly destructive to the economy. Yet, for instance, hempseed oil is legal in all 50 states and in over 40 countries, globally. Some fourteen states have laws on the books to add to this legality CBD oil, which is already legal for sale in Colorado, Washington, and Oregon. Additionally, there are millions of hemp oil consumers around the world, along with, now, additional millions of cannabis extract consumers. It is a number which is continuously rising based upon the plethora of research studies, plus compelling case histories, proving the medicinal powers of these novel substances.

Can anyone imagine it? All this potential is being resisted, economic capacities are being blocked, and, thus, vast opportunities are lost? The rest of the world takes advantage of it, greatly boosting their economic status, and, still, the United States loses out? Industrial hemp, the type used for making hard goods, such as car door frames, ropes, sails, textiles, paper, and detergent, along with highly nutritious seed oil, is no longer a commercial crop in America. It is now known that the plant can readily be converted into alcohol, to such a large degree that it could be created into a vehicle fuel. Industrial hemp contains only minimal amounts of THC, a mere 1.5% at the maximum and usually far less, as little as 0.2%. In contrast, the drug form contains some 5% to 10%, up to 10-fold greater or more.

The blockade by federal agencies is clearly a plot. The fact is industrial hemp, *Cannabis sativa*, has a long history of use in the Americas. In fact, in the early American colonies it was mandated that the colonists grow the crop for threat of fines and punishment by the British. Plus, in Victorian times extracts of cannabis were freely used as drugs with positive results.

Since the 1950s there has been an intensive scam against hemp. At that time it was put in the same category as the drug form. This doomed the plant as a crop item into virtual oblivion. This is despite the fact that industrial hemp is entirely different than the drug type. It is from a different species and biotype, essentially a subspecies, and the differences are significant. Even so, no one would smoke it. In fact, it would take dozens, perhaps, hundreds of cigarettes made from this type of hemp to get even a remote degree of psychoactive reactions. No one would do so.

It is a difference in cultivars. The reason the THC content in such hemp is so low is related to the resin. While naturally high in the psychoactive type it is low in the industrial one. The resin is a production of the buds and flowers of the female version of the plant. Industrial hemp is not cultivated to produce buds. What's more, this type of the plant has higher concentrations of other types of cannabinoids, notably cannabidiol, which antagonizes THC. There are other notable differences. The crop type has a highly crucial growth pattern, where it grows straight up rather than out laterally. Marijuana is incapable of growing in such a straight up fashion.

The upward growth is a sign of the crop's power and strength. Similar to bamboo, it contains fiber, a woody-like material, that has vast potential in industry and production. It can even be used to build furniture. No doubt, bamboo has become exceedingly popular. Hemp is the Northern Hemisphere's bamboo-like crop. What a dire shame that only corruption rules and that hemp is not grown nationally. After all, it is an economically invaluable crop. In fact, it is such an economic powerhouse that its free growth would essentially revolutionize America, causing it to have a thriving economy. Instead, the American population spends endless money obstructing it, preventing its farmers from capitalizing on it. In a further hypocrisy additional money must be spent, in fact, funds that it doesn't have, importing virtually all hemp goods, including hempseed oil and protein, when it could be grown more economically at home.

What a criminal act it is that the federal government systematically obstructs this industry. By doing so it has done vast damage to the American economy beyond any possible measure. Then, clearly, this government serves no useful function on behalf of the American people but, rather, acts as an antagonist: a truly corrupt element.

Thus, how can its position regarding hemp be held as credible? Regarding CBD oil the FDA has taken a virtual draconian position. In some of its opinions it has claimed that there is no place for cannabidiol-based supplements in the dietary supplement industry and that, specifically, CBD cannot be sold as a nutritional supplement. It has further mandated that cannabidiol-based supplements cannot be sold for another bizarre reason, which is that, essentially, 'We were first.' Yes, it is true the FDA has stated that its being first to the market with cannabidiol drugs is reason to mandate against CBD supplements.

Yet, CO_2 extracts are in a different league than CBD. These extracts are merely foods. Plus, the whole food type is not merely a CBD supplement but is, rather, a complex of 450-plus hemp-derived components, the most notable of which are the caryophyllenes, which are in a raw state, all of which are entirely safe for human consumption. Moreover, this extract, fortified with raw CO_2 oregano complex, is the only raw, unheated, and non-solvent extracted hemp stalk extract available. The rawness is crucial, since as a result the terpenes are highly maleable and are, thus, readily able to cross the blood-brain barrier. In one recent case history it was reported that a man with Lyme-induced tremors responded dramatically, with all tremors eliminated after taking the complex, as sublingual drops. This is a result of the great action of the raw terpenes in entering the brain tissue where they bind to the CB2 receptors, inducing brain cell regeneration.

No one has made Beta-caryophyllene, the primary active ingredient of cannabis, illegal. The substance and its derivatives are commonly used in the food processing industry, largely as a flavor additive. In this respect they are listed by the FDA as GRAS, that is Generally Regarded as Safe. Thus, Beta-caryophyllene-based dietary supplements are clearly legal, if not encouraged. It would be a crime against humanity to target Beta-caryophyllene-based supplements, just because they are from hemp. Despite this, the FDA's position is that it cannot be sold as a dietary supplement. Nor can any dietary supplement claims be made regarding it. Says the agency, essentially, cannabis drugs were first. This is through what it claims is investigational new drug application (IND). Further, the Drug Enforcement Administration (DEA) considers CBD a marijuana derivative, thus, from a federal point of view CBD oil is technically a Schedule 1 listed drug. Yet, this is complicated by the fact that some 14 states have made it legal to administer the herbal extract. Even so, it has never provided proof for its claim. In other words, the FDA has only one objective, which is to keep industrial hemp extract off the market in favor of sweetheart deals with drug makers. The wild oregano-hemp complex isn't a CBD supplement but is, rather, a caryophyllene and terpene extract.

Chapter Fifteen

Hemp and a Long Life

Can hemp influence lifespan? It is so nutritionally dense it would make sense that this is the case. Even so, when studying the plant, a hint is given. It is one of the longest existing commercial crops known. Moreover, the plant itself is tough and sturdy: tall-growing and disease resistant. This may give a clue regarding its lifespan-enhancing capacity. A recent study has determined that the key hemp active ingredient, Beta-caryophyllene, is a potent lifespan-promoting agent. The test model for longevity involves a tiny worm, the nematode, *Caenorhabditis elegans*. This small worm has been studied for years, because scientists can use it to model the potential for humans. In this breaking study the compound's ability to reduce stress is sufficiently powerful to increase the lifespan of this test worm, which means it has potential for human beings.

One other proof of Beta-caryophyllene's potential for a longer life relates to its ability to prevent substance abuse. In a

2014 study it was found that the substance reduced voluntary intake of alcohol by mice. This caused it to be recommended for treatment of alcoholism. Caryophyllene is an important antioxidant. Antioxidants are free radical scavengers that roam the body getting rid of damaging free radicals. By blocking or slowing down the free radical-induced effects of aging, Beta-caryophyllene promotes a longer life.

It appears that the molecule has greater powers than standard antioxidants, which have not shown dramatically obvious results in studies. While antioxidants failed to work with the nematode, Beta-caryophyllene did and did so dramatically.

One reason for the failure of standard antioxidants relates to their molecular or chemical nature. Rather than natural molecules, like caryophyllene, they are drugs: mere chemical imitations.

In many respects it appears as if the entire purpose of the hemp plant is to nourish the body in a most profound way. It was created for this purpose. Few if any plants can meet its diverse nutritional density. The leaf matter, seeds, and expressed seed oil, as well as protein, are all highly nourishing. It is, thus, an important source of food for human nutrition. Its deeper purpose is to support brain and nerve function through providing those rare dietary substances, the cannabinoids. It is as if it was created specifically for the body's endocannabinoid system.

Dangers of heat-treated hemp

For long, healthy life the benefits of hemp are found in the raw complexes. The application of heat greatly alters the chemistry of the delicate compounds in hemp, including the so-called diol compounds, along with the terpenes. It is heat which creates compounds with psychoactive powers as well as addictive powers. As well, Beta-caryophyllene is readily corrupted by heat and is most potent in the raw state. In this regard it should be realized that in many ways hemp is a green plant. Consider how dramatic the alteration in spinach or lettuce is if it is cooked. There is no comparison between the two, whether in flavor or appearance. For instance, raw lettuce is therapeutic to the body and is a good tonic for the stomach and intestines, while cooked lettuce has almost no such properties.

Delicate terpenes destroyed by heat and chemicals

Terpenes is the biologically active terpenes which largely account for hemp's therapeutic powers. These terpenes include Beta-caryophyllene, alpha pinene, linalool, myrcene, and limonene. All these terpenes are well-established aids to nervous system function, acting as relaxants, anticonvulsants, analgesics, and antiinflammatory agents. It merely demonstrates the vast powers of nature, all found in crude, raw extract of hemp leaves and stalk. All such terpenes are common components of herbs and spices, for instance, limonene, being a common constituent of citrus. Pinene is also readily found in nature, being one of the main terpenes in pine trees, sage, and rosemary.

Though they are less dense in quantity than the more complex Beta-caryophyllene and cannabinoids, the terpenes are essential components of the hemp medicine. These terpenes are the active ingredients of a number of other healthy, medicinal foods and spices such as citrus, lemongrass, pine, fir, sage, cumin, hops, and rosemary. They

234 The Cannabis Cure

have the novel capacity of readily penetrating the tissues, making their way directly into the cells, also having the ability to pass through the blood-brain barrier. Similar to petroleum products, terpenes are highly volatile. According to Raber extraction methods are a key issue in their preservation. If that extraction involves heating the plant matter, it is the terpenes which suffer the most, not the more complex cannabinoids. Heat, he says, typically destroys the terpenes, which evaporate at much lower temperatures than THC. Therefore, in order to achieve complete cannabis nutrition, raw, unheated extracts must be consumed. In this way the delicate, volatile, highly biologically active terpenes are preserved.

Nutritional value

The majority of the nutritional value in hemp is found in the seeds, the seed oil, and the fresh greens. Regarding the greens it is the expressed juice which is most dense and most easy to consume. This is in order to gain the full nutritional profile of the plant. However, such a juice is not readily available, while other forms, such as the seeds and seed oil, along with dry protein powder, are plentiful.

Let us begin with the seed oil. This oil is highly digestible. It provides the ideal ratio of omega 3s to omega 6s at 3:1. In addition, it is high in that rare omega 6 oil, GLA or gamma linolenic acid, the one found in primrose and borage oils. GLA is essential for cardiac, endocrine, and immune function. In fact, the oil is well established for its role in balancing hormone function. It is also an antidote for certain illnesses, notably migraines, fibromyalgia, intestinal disorders, nerve inflammation, and neurological complaints.

Regarding protein, hemp seeds are virtually a complete food, providing all nine essential amino acids. These are the substances required by the body on a daily basis for repairing damaged tissue and also to bolster hormone and neurological functions. This is why hemp seeds and hemp seed proteins are regarded as the perfect protein foods. The seeds, as well as the green matter, are rich in a special kind of protein known as soluble protein, which aids in elimination and also in blood sugar balance.

The vitamin-mineral content of hemp seeds is particularly impressive. They are a dense source of niacin, containing some 3 mg per 100 grams and also contain considerable amounts of other B vitamins, including vitamin B_1, riboflavin, and vitamin B_6. Regarding minerals, hemp seeds are a true nutritional powerhouse, containing dense amounts of calcium, magnesium, iron, phosphorus, manganese, potassium, and zinc. The content of magnesium and zinc is particularly impressive, with some 490 mg per 100 grams and 7 mg per 100 grams, respectively. The seeds also contain vitamin E as well as a plant form of vitamin D, the latter being only rarely found in vegetable matter.

Hemp fiber: the future

Hemp fiber is the longest, strongest and most durable of all natural fibers known. Hemp cultivation requires virtually no chemicals, pesticides or herbicides. Grown in rotation with other crops, such as corn and legumes, hemp farming is completely sustainable. The plant produces four times as much fiber per acre as pine trees. Hemp paper can be recycled up to seven times, compared with only three times for wood-pulp based papers. Hemp is easy to grow, and actually conditions soil wherever it grows. The seed and seed oil are rich in protein, essential fatty acids, and vitamins. Hemp is an ideal source of biomass for fuel. For instance, hemp ethanol burns cleanly and is the least polluting of all combustible fuel, even more so than biodiesel.

Hemp and humanity have been linked for over 10,000 years. It was humankind's first agricultural crop, remaining perhaps the planet's largest and most industrially important crop until the 19th century. No one smoked industrial hemp ever for purposes of getting high. There was no reason to destroy the industry. It was US- and European-based monopolistic families, like the DuPonts and the Hearsts, who destroyed it, merely for their own financial gain. This caused immeasurable loss in both economic and health realms for the Americas. In contrast, most of the non-Western world never stopped growing hemp, and today it is still commercially grown in China, Hungary, England, Canada, Australia, France, Italy, Spain, Holland, Germany, Poland, Romania, the Netherlands, Russia, Ukraine, Turkey, and India.

America, with its disabled economy, is denied this. Yet, what a catastrophe it is. Industrial hemp could transform the economy of the United States in a positive and beneficial way. Therefore, it should be exploited to its fullest potential. Only a massive public action against the autocratic government could achieve this. The corrupt government will never do so on its own.

Cold climates make the best hemp natural medicines

The finest quality hemp for the production of natural medicines is not the type grown in, for instance, the Deep

South or Mexico. Instead, it derives from colder climates often of higher elevation. THC-producing Marijuana must be grown in generally warm and humid environments. This is in order to produce the desired quantity and quality of THC-containing buds. However, since industrial hemp does not contain these buds, and the hardier parts of the plant are the more readily desired, it can be grown in a wider range of areas. The upper Midwest, the Rocky Mountain Areas, the Pacific Northwest, Northern Europe, and the South or North of Canada are ideal regions for such growth.

Cold-pressed hempseed oil: health food supreme

There is much nutrition and great therapeutic power in cold-pressed hemp seed oil. This is because it is a naturally rich source of those crucial nutritional components known as essential fatty acids. The oil is a dense source of healthy omega 6 fatty acids but also contains a considerable amount of omega 3s in a ratio of 3:1. Plus, it contains fatty acid rarely found in plant matter, docosahexaenoic acid or DHA, the same compound found in fish oils. This means it is excellent for brain health and is, thus, a healthy addition to the diet of infants, children, breast-feeding mothers, and pregnant women. DHA, in particular, is essential for normal development of the brain and retina during the first year of life and during the last trimester of pregnancy.

It is also beneficial for the skin as well as hair and scalp. In fact, these systems readily degenerate in the event of essential fatty acid deficiency. Consumed internally, it aids in the reversal of many skin abnormalities, including excessive oilinesss or dryness, as itchiness of the scalp, dandruff, hair loss, ringworm, mild eczema, and dermatitis. This may be in part due to its rich content of gamma linolenic acid and also DHA. It is a bona fide medicine in its own right. Consider its actions on the cardiovascular system. In one study published by Hungarian investigators it was found to have a modest effect in reversing degenerative disease of the arteries. Regarding skin conditions an evaluation of the benefit of hempseed oil versus olive oil was conducted. The investigators publishing in the *Journal of Dermatological Treatment* found that hempseed oil significantly "improved clinical symptoms of atopic dermatitis" more effectively than olive oil. This is fully a result of the rich array of biologically active polyunsaturated fatty acids in the oil.

In yet another investigation it was determined that in a rat model hempseed, in this case the entire seed, had profound effects on the heart muscle. As determined through ischemic imagery hearts from rats supplemented with the seed meal gained maximal contraction function of the heart muscle and also enhanced rates of muscle tension then relaxation during reperfusion greater than the hearts from control groups. This means that, essentially, the heart became a more effective relaxation-tension pump as a result of the hempseed intake.

These positive effects are largely a consequence of its dense content of alpha linolenic acid. This key fatty acid is involved in the production of a number of essential substances, notably those which act as cellular mediators: the prostaglandins.

Alpha linolenic acid is an essential nutrient, that is an essential fatty acid, which means it is critical to life itself.

Without it, the cells and organs of the body degenerate. Its not sufficient to merely consume the monounsaturates and the saturated fats. The body needs a certain amount of polyunsaturates for optimal health. Symptoms or conditions associated with alpha linolenic acid deficiency include hypertension, high blood triglyceride levels, sticky, thick blood, immune system disorders, obesity, slow metabolic rate, swelling, dry hair, dry skin, brittle or weak nails, dermatitis-like lesions, asthma, bronchitis, and mental deterioration. Conditions which respond to hempseed oil therapy are numerous. These conditions include arthritis, diabetes, cancer, eczema, dermatitis, psoriasis, high cholesterol, high triglycerides, hair loss, hardening of the arteries, heart disease, varicose veins, hormonal disorders, infertility, lung disorders, and obesity.

In many respects hempseed oil is a premier polyunsaturated fatty acid supplement. Not only does it contain healthy amounts of the relatively rare alpha linolenic acid, but it also contains its key metabolite, gamma linolenic acid. The other essential fatty acid, linoleic acid, is also found in dense amounts, but more rare is the fact that the oil contains linoleic acid's metabolite, too, stearidonic acid, which is rarely present in commercial oils. For instance, there is no such a substance in canola, corn, soy, sunflower, and/or olive oil; these oils are also deficient in GLA. Moreover, GLA is an essential nutrient upon which life itself is dependent. The tissues degenerate as a result of the deficiency, and this is true of a deficit in linoleic and linolenic acids as well.

It was seven-time Nobel Prize nominee J. Budwig who demonstrated the vast role of essential fatty acids in disease treatment and prevention. Her success included reversal of heart infarctions, arthritis, cancer, and other common diseases with rather large doses of these compounds. She related their powers to their abilities to do something phenomenal, which was to "store electrons from the sun," which is a critical factor for human health. Notes Budwig:

> The sun's rays are very much in harmony with humans. It is no coincidence that we love the sun. The resonance in our biological tissue is so strongly tuned to the absorption of solar energy that physicists who occupy themselves with the scientific phenomenon, the quantum biologists, say there is nothing on earth that has a higher concentration of solar energy photons than humans...

She added: "An abundance of these electrons, which are tuned to the solar frequency, exist...in many seed oils. Scientifically, these seed oils have been designated as electron-rich, essential, highly unsaturated fats."

Raw hempseed oil is merely trapped photonic energy, that is trapped sunlight, in the oil phase. Because it is so rich in electrons it has a tendency towards rancidity. Moreover, it is so sensitive to heat that it should never be used in cooking. It is relatively vulnerable to oxidation and, thus, must be refrigerated.

This is true of the typical cold-pressed oil. However, a more crude hempseed oil is now available made from the first crude, whole, unprocessed pressing. This is the first grade of hempseed oil, never filtered or refined. Fortified with antioxidant-rich spice oils, along with raw CO_2-extracted hemp oil, it is far more stable than the standard type. The spice, black seed, and hemp stalk extracts provide a litany of natural substances with therapeutic powers, including carvacrol, rosmarinic acid, Beta-caryophyllene, pinene, linalool, cannabinoids, thymoquinone, and limonene. The addition of such oils potentiates the powers of hempseed oil, while also causing its preservation, preventing it from going rancid. With this fortified power such an oil becomes even more potent for cardiac, skin, and immune health, while also acting as a powerful internal cleanse.

Hemp protein to the rescue

Hemp seeds are among the most nutritionally dense of all foods. For thousands of years they have held a high status as a nutritional source. For instance, in Ottoman Turkey hemp seeds were used as a protein source to aid in the recovery of people stricken by serious diseases.

It's not even a true seed but is, rather, technically, a nut, which demonstrates the immensity of its nutritional powers. The seed itself contains a dense amount of oil at some 30%. No wonder migrating birds relish in it. Regarding the protein density it is also exceedingly high at 25%.

The two main proteins in hempseed are edestin and albumin. These highly digestible proteins are exceedingly high-quality, difficult to procure in any other vegetable food. Because of the rich amount of the albumin, the consumption of hempseed protein is essential for those suffering from chronic, degenerative diseases, including liver disorders, heart disease, and cancer. Deficiencies of albumin in the human body are common and quite disastrous. This is a crucial protein for aiding in the maintenance of fluid volume, also acting as a transporting agent for other nutrients.

Albumin is made in the liver, and a deficiency is a sign of a disorder of this organ. In fact, it is a vicious cycle, since a lack of this key protein causes the liver to continue to degenerate. This is why hempseed protein is an ideal type for liver cell regeneration.

For people of all ages it is readily digested and highly nutritious. For the weak and recovering patient it is an ideal addition to the nutritional protocol. A powerful, organic, raw hempseed protein powder is now available. Known as NutriHEMP raw it is fortified with organic, raw, sprouted brown rice protein this is a complete protein supplement with all 9 essential amino acids for human nutrition. It also contains wild, raw chaga and is sweetened merely with raw, organic yacon powder, which acts as a prebiotic and weight loss aid. In order to gain the benefits of hempseed protein take one or two heaping tablespoonsful of this protein powder in juice or in a smoothie daily or every other day. For body builders and sports-people who are highly active double or even triple this dose. Regular consumption of such a fortified hempseed protein powder decreases the appetite thereby facilitating weight loss. It may also be used for weight gain in athletic people through the addition of raw egg yolk, whole organic milk, and raw honey.

Hemp seeds as a food additive

It is commonplace, now, to find hemp seeds in the health food marketplace. What a positive issue it is, since these seeds are among the most nutritionally dense food complexes known.

For good health it is ideal to include them in the diet. The primary nutrients found in the seeds are protein and essential fatty acids. The seeds are also a top source of minerals, notably zinc, iron, and magnesium. Regarding the latter the density is significant. They are one of the few ultra-dense sources of magnesium, containing some 50% of the daily minimum in a mere 100 gram serving. The seeds are also rich in vitamin E, with a mere three tablespoons containing 20% of the daily need. Regarding carbohydrates hemp seeds are low, and so they make a great addition to a weight loss program. Because of their high amount of fat and protein, they are highly filling. Combined with other nuts/seeds, such as toasted sesame seeds and sunflower seeds, it becomes a complete protein additive.

Danger of synthetic cannabis

For good health and prevention of disease it is important to know of the dangerous types of 'cannabis,' for instance, the synthetic kinds often found in street drugs. There are also novel drugs based on cannabidiol, which are produced synthetically. A number of man-made cannabis substances have been approved for human use. In many respects the entire premise of such drug-like substances is erroneous. In most cases only a single cannabinoid chemical is produced, while in nature within cannabis there are many dozens of such compounds. By no means can a mere isolate or in this case lone synthetic substance replace the whole. Moreover, these compounds rather than promoting health ultimately corrupt it. One such substance was the drug Rimonabant. Originally, it was produced as an appetite-controlling drug or anti-obesity agent. Yet, shortly after its release it was withdrawn form the market because of serious side-effects, including fatality. Rimonabant, approved in Europe and other countries but not in the US, acts by blocking CB1

244 The Cannabis Cure

receptors. In other words, it effectively shuts down a goodly portion of th endocannabinoid system.

The side effects, though, were dramatic. People became depressed and also developed suicidal thoughts. A number of people committed suicide as a result of the drug, two in one town in Ireland alone. A number of others were admitted to the hospital for suicidal desires but were stabilized. One of the deaths was of a 22 year-old male, who hung himself. The deaths occurred in study participants, who paid up to 200 euros per week for the medication. There were also reports of anxiety, agitation, anger, delusions, a desire for self-harm, and psychosis. People trusted it, since it was related to the cannabis plant. That trust was lost, as some six people died from suicide alone.

The toxicity proved to be extreme. Routinely, it seemed to do the opposite of true, whole food CBD. Side effects included loss of appetite, tooth decay, exhaustion, apathy, tremors, insomnia, breathlessness, skin destruction, and heart conditions requiring medication.

In contrast, carbon dioxide-extracted hemp cannabinoids can never do this, inducing neither cardiac nor neurological failure. Even with marijuana this is rare, with overdoses from acute cardiac or respiratory failure being unheard of, especially in adults. This demonstrates the short-sighted thinking of turning natural herbs into patented drugs. Ironically, truly natural, whole food cannabis—the raw, complete CO_2 complex with all the cannabinoids and Beta-caryophyllene plus the aromatic compounds—does precisely the opposite. It halts any tendency for suicide and the propensity for self-harm, while it also prevents many of those symptoms induced by the drug: anxiety, agitation, tendency towards anger, psychosis, and delusions. There is no suicidal ideation with this natural medicine, in fact, precisely the opposite: the robust desire for more and more life. Yes, indeed, crude hemp extract with crude, raw oregano, both rich in healthy cannabinoids, obliterates such symptoms. Yet, it is true of all isolates and synthetics, that is in relation to cannabinoids. All have potential side effects which never occur in the crude, whole food, and raw, extract. Plus, the addition of wild, raw oregano extract creates a great balance in the chemistry of hemp extract, leading to a superior formula. The nervous system is too delicate yet also too powerful in its capacities to be manipulated: without risk of dire consequences:

Texas Man High on Synthetic Marijuana Kills and Eats Neighbor's Dog

ICTMN Staff, June 26, 2012

Synthetic marijuana, known as "spice" and "K-2," is being blamed for a horrific story in Waco, Texas, in which 22-year-old Michael Terron Daniel strangled, then began to eat, a neighbor's dog, who died at the scene.

Officers found Daniel sitting on the porch covered in blood and was "initially incoherent and unresponsive," said Waco police Sgt. W. Patrick Swanton, and was taken to Providence Health Center. While waiting for paramedics to arrive, Swanton said, Daniel asked officers to fight him or use a stun gun "to help him get off his bad trip," though officers did neither. Spice is thought to exacerbate existing neuroses.

This is the consequence of synthesizing or semi-synthesizing single cannabinoids, likely tainted with various contaminants. Such isolated compounds strike with too vigorous of an impact, creating serious imbalances within cortical function. What is the body to do? It is used in nature to a different exposure; the whole complex of dozens of cannabinoids and related molecules: all at once. In this case the drugs, illicit or otherwise, overload the system, and the consequences are unpredictable. Even so, with actual marijuana such highly violent occurrences are relatively rare, but they can and do occur, especially with THC-fortified varieties. In this regard it must be kept in mind that cannabis contains over 60 cannabinoids and some 450 active ingredients. How can the ingestion of a single one of these ingredients alone cause anything other than an imbalance?

The power of signal control

Perhaps the most novel aspect of cannabis as a role player in a long, healthy life relates to its regulatory powers. It is most incredible, but it is true. Food has the power to regulate or normalize the body through its influence on the nervous system. What are the most powerful of these foods? It is those which contain the signalling agents, the cannabinoids and related molecules.

If the nervous system is unable to send signals, its functions collapse. When this happens, a wide range of symptoms develop, including neurological, immunological, and cardiac ones. The ability to handle stress is diminished. There is depression and anxiety. There is poor mood, irritability, agitation, and even a lack of desire or happiness. When this happens, the propensity for drug addiction rises.

These are all symptoms of cannabinoid deficiency particularly common in those who fail to consume cannabinoid-rich foods and spices.

With failure of the inter-communication systems there are consequences. Cell growth is stalled. Toxins accumulate. The ability of the cells and organs in self-repair is obstructed. There is no means for the body to renew itself: that is in the event of endocannabinoid failure. This may explain the astounding finding that the all-important dietary component cannabinoid Beta-caryophyllene in particular causes an extension of lifespan in laboratory studies. It's divine—biblical, too. No wonder the parsley, sage, rosemary, and thyme (actually, wild oregano) consumers in the Mediterranean live longer than the non-consumers.

Thus, the key to a long, vigorous life is optimal inter-neuron signaling. This is precisely the domain of the cannabinoids. Through the regular intake of these compounds nervous system function can be restored. This demonstrates the importance of adding natural cannabinoid sources to the daily regimen. Such sources include black pepper, cinnamon, cloves, cumin, rosemary, sage, thyme, wild oregano, hempseeds, hempseed oil, olives, and extra virgin olive oil. It also demonstrates the crucial need to take, supplementally, the wild oregano-hemp CO_2 complex, along with spice oil-fortified hempseed oil, and supplements containing wild rosemary, wild sage, cinnamon, and cloves: or their oil extracts. With clove oil make sure it is clove bud oil, not the leaf oil, the latter being inedible. For a wide range of Beta-caryophyllene-rich supplements and extracts see www.americanwildfoods.com.

Chapter Sixteen

Conclusion

Is it not bizarre? On the one hand hemp is a powerful natural medicine yet in another form it can be hallucinogenic and can even ultimately corrupt the overall health. Few plants have such a double power. Most plants which act as medicines have no such dual effects. Alcohol cannot be compared. It is not an herb or a plant complex but is, rather, a bacterial ferment and is a poison outright. Tobacco is closer to this, in fact, the most extreme example. The original, native forms of tobacco were herbal and were used by the aboriginal people, medicinally. In the Western world its use was first realized upon observing natives in Cuba and Haiti smoking it. The smoke was held a panacea, largely for germ infections. This makes sense, since the active ingredient of tobacco, nicotine, is toxic to all cells. The raw, whole plant or its extract was also found effective at wound healing, notably versus abscesses, fistulas, and infected sores. It was used mainly in desperate cases but was deemed so effective that it was called "Holy Herb." The plant was also used in the form of the fresh green leaves, breathing the odor, for headaches.

This is the nature of God's medicine. In certain forms virtually all plants are medicinal. Even poison hemlock was used in medieval times as a medicine for certain disorders (not advisable today, though).

With native use it was the matter of using basically an unprocessed, whole plant. Side effects and toxicity were relatively rare.

This is surely not the case today; that is, no one uses the herbal form, only the pre-made drug agent. The tobacco plant is responsible for a greater number of deaths than any other herb. As described by A. Charlton in *Medicinal Uses of Tobacco in History*, currently, tobacco smoking causes some three million deaths world-wide, which is catastrophic. No other toxin can remotely compare to the destruction it causes. If nothing is done about this, by 2030, it is predicted, some 10 million total will die yearly. No other substance abuse causes such a massive amount of catastrophic, premature deaths. This is the Old World's curse from the New World, make no mistake about it. Instead of the Old World adopting the methods of the natives, which was the use of the whole, unprocessed plant, it was corrupted by turning tobacco smoking into a highly destructive profit system. With marijuana there is also profiteering, in this case by not only professional and amateur drug dealers but also the federal government through its trumped-up war on drugs.

Even so, consider the hypocrisy of the so-called drug wars. No one bans the consumption of, for instance, tobacco or alcohol. No one arrests youths for gathering on their own in legal domains and drinking endless amounts of alcohol or smoking tobacco, virtually until the room turns blue: even though it is dangerous and will likely hurt the users and also innocent others. It has all been corrupted by great power brokers, the powerful ones of vested interests: all to protect their wretched monopolies. For instance, the DuPont family proved highly malicious, destroying the hemp industry to protect its own synthetic productions, such as nylon, while that other criminal clique, the Hearst family, did so to protect lumber and paper interests. Federal laws were put in place to protect such vested interests. Even today, the free use of industrial hemp poses a threat to the monopolists. Thus, there is no realistic approach to marijuana, and as a result, its greatness languishes.

Yet, there is legitimate concern about the promotion of marijuana as a recreational agent. There is no benefit to smoking any substance recreationally. This should be discouraged, especially daily or weekly use, but this does not mean users should be subjected to draconian punishment, like ridiculously long prison sentences.

What about those who sell the agent? That approach, too, is fatally skewed. How can the degree of punishment be justified? A significant fine and community service, perhaps counseling, would make far more sense. Now, it is legal in some areas to smoke pot as well as eat it, also grow it. Yet, currently, there are people in prison who may even die there for selling the drug.

Consider the fate of a homeless man of Shreveport Louisiana, Mr. F. V. Winslow. Set up, he was approached by an undercover cop seeking to buy pot. After selling him two crumpled bags for a mere $10 each he found himself in a squad car. Winslow was found guilty of selling a Schedule I Controlled Dangerous Substance. As reported in *Mother Jones Magazine,* he was given *life in prison with no chance for parole.* The man should be released from prison immediately. He was set up via a plot, and the punishment meted out was extreme, fully draconian.

For the mere crime of pot trade the punishment of life beyond bars is hard to fathom. Yet, this is far from unique, with some 70 other marijuana sellers in the US imprisoned for life. Government powerful ones participate in the orchestration of illicit wars, causing the deaths of tens of thousands, even millions, of people. Yet, these individuals, fully publically known, are given a free pass? Moreover, yearly, a greater number of people are arrested for pot possession than all violent crimes combined. Pot is the target, but the murderers, embezzlers, thieves, and rapists are not? The punishment against pot smoking and its sellers itself is a condemnable racket.

Thus, a sound approach needs to be established to wade through this, to make sense between propaganda and reality. This is through the full legalization of the non-hallucinogenic types of marijuana, usable *Cannabis sativa,* the so-called industrial marijuana. No doubt, a whole food, raw extract of hemp, one free of all chemicals and toxins, is an ideal adjunct to good health. It can only do good, that is there is no way it can cause any harm. Then why is it banned for human consumption to any degree?

Yet, how can sanity ever prevail in the United States? It is corrupt beyond belief, so overwhelmed by vested interests: so skewed by those greedy ones who hold power. Through government, that is federal, policy it is unlikely that this substance will ever achieve a balanced, legitimate status. There is only one way to do so. It is the people who must drive this revolution. It is human intelligence that can change this. It can all change through education and consumer demand. Insanely long prison sentences are not the answer. It must start in the schools, whether private or public. Youths must be educated about the danger of intoxicants, not only marijuana but also alcohol, opiates, and tobacco. They should be taught about the danger of using street drugs and the potential for contamination. They should be given options besides drug abuse for enjoyment and elevation of mood. Nutritional knowledge should be instilled, since sound nutrition is the great defense against substance abuse.

The historical use of these substances should be taught. So should, historically, the danger and benefits of their use be explained. For instance, in the 1800s the Chinese were turned into opium addicts. What good did it do for them? Families should be exposed to the danger of these three most prominently abused intoxicants. Simultaneously, the medicinal properties of marijuana, rather, cannabis, should be explored and realized.

What should be done about the much sought-after options of marijuana smoking? Medical use should be under a doctor's management. To self medicate with any harsh drug, whether codeine, cocaine, or marijuana, can prove dangerous, as it can lead to addiction. At this point the addict is left to the self. No one can predict what will happen to such a one. In particular, the extremely potent type, hashish, is unfit for human consumption as a recreational agent. It should only be used as a medical treatment under a doctor's care: period.

Marijuana, though, is used as an excuse to ban all forms of cannabis, even the intoxication-free, medicinal type. This is a great detriment to the human race. This is being done exclusively to protect vested interests. Let the public demand make it clear that the United States is against the monopolistic war against industrial hemp. In this regard vast profits are being lost that would benefit the people-at large. Let the US states consider all issues, including the excessively extreme punishments against pot smoking and/or its sale. Thus, let there be an entirely new approach, one based on thorough knowledge and common sense, based upon the obvious benefits to humankind. Let it be an educational approach, the awareness method, the one that will save the country and its youth from further damage and from adopting substance abuse as a means of mood elevation, even rebellion.

Moreover, with an organized effort it can be done. The world can explore just what causes people to turn to hallucinogens. It is surely a lack of peace in the heart. It is also a lack of kindness, generosity, and, particularly, love. All people could get involved in this. Organizations for just this purpose could be started. A true, legitimate war, rather, campaign, could be initiated, the campaign against senseless human harm. It is the harm which occurs when people fill their lives with the dangerous, addictive substances of nature, the habit-forming acts of pot smoking, cocaine use, heroin injection, tobacco smoking, alcohol consumption, and more.

It is the people themselves who commit these acts: with their own two hands. Moreover, it is never done for 'health' purposes. Thus, the question must be asked, "Why has society fallen to this level? What has caused people to do this? What is missing from their lives?" The heart-felt love for God is one factor. This is not to preach, but it is a certain fact. The deep, profound faith in this almighty Being is one of the most powerful elements conceivable. This is for bringing the deepest levels of peace within the heart: for each person's benefit, not for that of the creator.

It is time, now, to make a difference, to change the course, and to put a halt to it all. It is time to stop the self-destruction of human beings by their own actions. This is through curtailing the use of all addictive substances, which do much to harm and do nothing to aid. Instead, let the plants—the herbs, spices, foods, and more—of the Creative Being be the source for all that benefits human kind. Among these most astounding sources are whole, unaltered, fully natural extracts of medicinal oregano. Yet another is that ultra-sophisticated, incredibly versatile raw CO_2 extract of organically grown *Cannabis sativa*, the most ideal natural medicine for the support of the nervous system, the immune system, digestive wellness, and far more. Raw Beta-caryophyllene, found in dense amounts in these extracts, is the natural medicine of the future. Take advantage of it for a powerful, long-lasting improvement in overall health.

Appendix A

Conditions which respond to CO_2 hemp-wild oregano therapy

Neurological

Alzheimer's disease/dementia

multiple sclerosis

Parkinson's disease and ALS

depression

anxiety/nervous agitation

epilepsy and other seizure syndromes

post-traumatic stress syndrome

post-stroke recovery syndrome

schizophrenia

obsessive-compulsive syndrome

autism/ADD

brain damage and/or coma

suicidal ideation

tremors

insomnia

sleep apnea

memory loss

post-encephalitis syndrome

paralysis

Digestive/intestinal

pancreatitis
cirrhosis of the liver
hepatitis
esophageal varices
esophagitis
gastritis
GERD
gastric ulcer
duodenal ulcer
irritable bowel syndrome/colitis
ulcerative colitis
Crohn's disease
spastic colon
nausea/vomiting

Lung/bronchial

emphysema
COPD
bronchitis
asthma
chronic cough

Immune/autoimmune

cancer of all types, including leukemia and lymphoma
low white count
immune deficiency syndrome
Lyme disease
intestinal parasitism

Joint, muscular, and inflammatory

fibromyalgia

polymyositis

arthritis

Lyme disease

plantar fasciitis

rheumatoid arthritis

bursitis

spinal disorders, including spinal stiffness

ankylosing spondylitis

chronic pain

bone disease

Other

alcohol, tobacco, and drug addiction

addiction to mood-altering agents such as SSRIs

glaucoma

retinal detachment

macular degeneration

floaters

diabetes

chemotherapy/radiation damage

adrenal exhaustion

heart/circulatory disease

sugar addiction

chronic pain syndromes

migraine headaches

high stress syndrome

Bibliography

Al-Khalifa, A., et al. 2007. Effect of dietary hempseed intake on cardiac ischemia-reperfusion injury. *Am. J. Physiol. Regul. Integr. Comp. Physiol.* 292:R1198-203.

Bento, A. F., et al. 2011Beta-Caryophyllene inhibits dextran sulfate sodium-induced colitis in mice through CB2 receptor activation and PPARy pathway. *Am. J. Pathol.* 178:1153

Bittencourt, P. R., Sander, J. W. and S. Mazer. 1999. Viral, bacterial, fungal, and parasitic infections associated with seizure disorders. In: Meinardi, H., ed., *Handbook of Clinical Neurology*, V: 72. Amsterdam: Elsevier Sciences.

Blaszczak-Boxe, A. 2015. *Marijuana May Trigger Allergies in Some People.* LiveScience. Mar. 06, www.livescience.com/50059-marijuana-allergies.html.

Boysen, S. R., et al. 2002. Tremorgenic mycotoxicosis in four dogs from a single household. *J. Am. Vet. Med. Assoc.* 221:1441.

Callaway, J., Schwab, U., Harvima, I., et al. 2005. Efficacy of dietary hempseed oil in patients with atopic dermatitis. *J. Dermatolog. Treatment.* 16:87.

Consroe, P., Carlini, E. A. Zwicker, A. P. and L. Al Lacerda. 1979. Interaction of cannabidiol and alcohol in humans. *Psychopharmacology.* 66:45-50.

Devinsky, O., Thiele, E, Laux, L., et al. 2015. Efficacy and safety of Epidiolex (cannabidiol) in children and young adults with treatment-resistant epilepsy: update from the expanded access program. *Amer. Epil. Soc. Annual Meeting Abstracts. Abstract* 3.397.

Drysdale, A. J. and B. Platt. 2003. Cannabinoids: mechanisms and therapeutic applications in the CNS. *Curr. Med. Chem.* 10:2719.

El-Remessy, A.B., et al. 2003. Neuroprotective effect of (-)Delta9-tetrahydrocannabinol and cannabidiol in N-methyl-D-aspartate-induced retinal neurotoxicity: involvement of peroxynitrite. *Am. J. Pathol.* 163:1997-2008.

Eskay, R., et al. 2005. Cannabidiol, antioxidants, and diuretics in reversing binge ethanol-induced neurotoxicity. *American Soc. Pharcol. Exp. Ther.*

Fernandez-Ruiz, J., Sagredo, O., Pazos, M. R., Garcia, C., Pertwee, R., Mechoulam, R., and J. Martinez-Orgado. 2013. Cannabidiol for neurodegenerative disorders: important new clinical applications for this phytocannabinoid? *Br. J. Clin. Pharm.* 75:323.

Fernandez-Ruiz, J., Moro, M. A., and J. Martinez-Orgado. 2015. Cannabinoids in neurodegenerative disorders and stroke/brain trauma: from preclinical models to clinical applications. *Neurotherapeutics.* 12: 793.

Gertsch, J., Leonti, M., Raduner, S., Racz, I., and J. Chen, et al. 2008. Beta-Caryophyllene is a dietary cannabinoid. *Proc. Natl. Acad. Sci.* 105:9099-9104.

Gilling, D. H., et al. 2014. Antiviral efficacy and mechanisms of action of oregano essential oil and its primary component carvacrol against murine norovirus. *J. Appl. Microbiol.* 116:1149-1163.

Hancock-Allen, J. B., et al. 2015. Notes from the field: death following ingestion of an edible marijuana product, Colorado, March 2014. MMWR.

Hartley, J. P., et al. 1978. Bronchodilator effect of delta-1-tetrahydrocannabinol. *Br. J. Clin. Pharmacol.* 5:523-525.

Jouanjus, E., et al. 2014. Marijuana use may increase heart complications in young, middle-aged adults. *Journal of American Heart Association* (online version, April)

Klein, T. W. and C. A. Newton. 2007. Therapeutic potential of cannabinoid-based drugs. *Adv. Exp. Med. Biol.* 601:395.

Koultroumanidou, E. 2013. Increased seizure latency and decreased severity of pentylenetetrazol-induced seizures in mice after essential oil administration. *Epilepsy Res. Treat.* 2013: 532657.

Lachenmeier, D. and J. Rehm. Marijuana vs. Alcohol: Which is Really Worse for Your Health? *Scientific Reports.* 5:8126.

Melis, M. and M. Pistis. 2007. Endocannabinoid signaling in midbrain dopamine neurons: more than physiology? *Curr. Neuropharmacol.* 5:268-277.

Michler, T., Storr, M., Kramer, J., Ochs, S., Malo, A., Reus, S., Goke, B., and C. Schafer. 2013. Activation of cannabinoid receptor 2 reduces inflammation in acute experimental pancreatitis via intra-acinar activation of p38 and MK2-dependent mechanisms. *Am. J. Physiol. Gastrointest. Liver Physiol.* 15:G181.

Mir, A., Obafemi, A., Young, A., and C. Kane. 2011. Myocardial infarction associated with the use of synthetic cannabinoid K2. *Pediatrics.* 128(6).

Mittleman, M. A., et al. 2001. Triggering myocardial infarction by marijuana. *Circulation.* 103:2805.

Nahas, G. Hashish in Islam 9th to 18th Century. *Bull. N.Y. Acad. Med.*

Nargarkatti, P., Pandey, R., Rieder, S. A., Hegde, V. L. and M. Nagarkatti. Cannabinoids as novel anti-inflammatory drugs. *Future Med. Chem.* 1: 1333.

Pacher, P., Sandor, B., and G. Kunos. 2006. The endocannabinoid system as an emerging target of pharmacotherapy. *Pharmacol Rev.* 58:389–462.

Pacher, P. and S. Steffens. 2009. The emerging role of the endocannabinoid system in cardiovascular disease. *Semin. Immunopathol.* 31:63-77.

Rezkaila, S. H., Shrma, P., and R. A. Korner. 2003. Coronary no-flow and ventricular tachycardia associated with habitual marijuana use. *Forensic Sci. Int.* 42:365.

Sagredo, O, et. al. 2011. Neuroprotective effects of phytocannabinoid-based medicines in experimental models of Huntington's disease. *J. Neurosci. Res.* 89:1509.

Sander, J. W. Infectious Agents and Epilepsy. In: *The Infectious Etiology of Chronic Diseases: Defining the Relationship, Enhancing the Research, and Mitigating the Effects* - Workshop Summary.

Smith, C. G. and R. H. Asch. 1984. Acute, short-term, and chronic effects of marijuana on the female primate reproductive function. *NIDA Res. Monogr.* 44:82-96.

Taylor, L., et al. 2015. Primary macrophage chemotaxis induced by cannabinoid receptor 2 agonists occurs independently of the CB2 receptor. *Sci. Rep.* 5:10682.

Tomida, I., Azuara-Blanco, A., House, H., Flint, M., Pertwee, R. G., and P. J. Robson. 2006. Effect of sublingual application of cannabinoids on intraocular pressure: a pilot study. *J. Glaucoma.* 15:349.

Toson, El-Shahat A. 2011. Impact of marijuana smoking on liver and sex hormones: Correlation with oxidative stress. *Nature & Science.* 9:76.

Varner, M. W., et al. 2013. Association Between Stillbirth and Illicit Drug Use and Smoking During Pregnancy. *Obstetrics & Gynecology.*

Wagner, J. A., Abesser, M., Karcher, J., Laser, M. and G. Kunos 2005. Coronary vasodilator effects of endogenous cannabinoids in vasopressin-preconstricted unpaced rate ioslated hearts. *J. Cardiovasc. Pharmacol.* 46:348.

Williams, S. J., Hartley, J. P., and J. D. Graham. 1976. Brochodislator effect of delta-1-tetrahydrocannabinol administered by aerosol of asthmatic patients. *Thorax.* 31:720.

Woodruff, A.W., Bisseru, B., and J.C. Bowe. 1966. Infection with animal helminths as a factor in causing poliomyelitis and epilepsy. *British Medical Journal.* 5503:1576

Internet sources:

http://www.hightimes.com/read/talking-terpenes

http://theleafonline.com/c/science/2014/10/terpene-profile-caryophyllene

http://hempethics.weebly.com/industrial-hemp-vs-cannabis.html

http://www.drugtext.org/Cannabis-marijuana-hashish/acute-and-chronic-toxicity-of-marijuana.html

Monitoring the Future study, 2013, Univ. of Michigan

Cannabis: Terpenes and Their Effects. Hemp Edification.
Hempedification.blogsot.com.

Index

A

Addiction
  alcohol, 91, 199
  drug, 91, 193, **199-201**, 246, 258
  marijuana, 48, 258
  sugar, 149, **203-204**, 258
  tobacco, **201-202**
  pot, 202-203
Adrenal exhaustion, 122, 125, **181-182**, 258
Adrenal glands, 11, 50, 58, 59, 122, 125, 157, 181, 182, 207
Alcoholism, 194, 200, 232
Allergy, 80, 81, 184
ALS, 91, 105, 113, **143-146**, 256
Alzheimer's disease, 91, 113, 256
Anxiety, 20, 21, 25, 49, 50, 73, 84, 90, 99, 100, 112, 116, 119, 128, **156-159**, 198, 203, 207, 244, 246, 256
Arthritis, 11, 22, 23, 91, 239, 240, 258
Asthma, 80, 140, **182-185**, 239, 257
Autism, 91, 109, 111, 113, **152-154**, 256
Autophagy, 27, 56

B

Basil, 9, 13, 14, 22, 23, 92-95, 106, 114, 118, 122, 127, 134-137, 155, 167, 175, 176, 179, 187

Baudelaire, Charles, 39, 40, 41
Beta-caryophyllene, 9-14, 18-24, 38, 54, 98, 114, 120, 122, 125, 135, 137, 141, 153, 154, 164, 167, 180, 185-191, 198, 208, 211, 212, 228, 231-233, 241, 244, 247, 255
  antiinflammatory actions of, 22
Black pepper, 9, 13, 14, 19, 22, 88, 92-95, 134, 135, 167, 175, 176, 180, 187, 206, 208, 247
Blood sugar, 122, 125, 155, 156, 159, 172, 178, 203, 204, 208, 235
Bone disease, **210-213**, 258
Brain damage, 74, 75, 89, 151, **164-166**, 256
Bronchitis, 140, 239, 257

C

Cancer, 11, 25, 28, 34, 72, 91, 95, 97, 100, 105, 113, 116, 153-154, **187-190**, 201, 211, 212, 223, 239-241, 257
Candida, 108, 124, 140, 149, 150, 155-157, 185,
Cannabidiol, 20, 21, 30, 31, 76, 97-102, 121, 132, 164, 167, 179, 188, 190, 221, 227, 228, 243
Cannabinoid deficiency test, **90-96**
Cannabis sativa, 226, 252, 255
Carbon monoxide, 59, 60, 84, 130
Cardiovascular system, 51, 83, 127, 238
Caryophyllene oxide, 20
CB1 receptors, 11, 19, 30, 63, 68, 69, 130, 177, 243-244
CB2 receptors, 11, 19, 20-22, **29-30**, 128, 177, 198, 211
CBD oil, **30-31**, 76, 97-103, 121, 131, 147, 154, 166, 181, 188, 197, 199, 219, 221, 225, 228, 229, 244

Chaga, 126, 127, 131, 134, 146, 148, 149, 154, 162, 163, 165, 166, 172, 191, 192, 203, 213, 242

Chemotherapy, 87, 126, 180, **190-192**, 258

Chronic cough, 38, 139, 257

Chronic depression, **155-156**

Chronic pain syndromes, 38, 42, 78, 91, 113, 123, 134-138, 258

CHS, 43

Cinnamon, 13, 14, 23, 94, 95, 117, 118, 124, 125, 127, 140, 154, 175, 178, 180, 185, 204, 206, 208, 247

Circulatory disease, 127, 258

Club des Hashischins, 40, 42

Cocaine, 19, 35, 54, 63, 68, 70, 77, 82, 193, 199, 201, 222, 253, 254

COPD, 139, 140, 201, 257

CO_2 hemp extract, 13, 105, 106, 122, 182, 208
 see also hemp

D

Dementia, 36, 91, 100, 112, 256

Depression, 50, 73, 91, 112,116, 128, 155, 156, 169, 188, 209, 216, 246, 256

Diabetes, 72, 100, **178-180**, 239, 258

Digestive disorders, 119, **175-176**

E

Emphysema, 140, 201, 257

Endocannabinoid system,9, 13, **26-29**, 55, 57, 77, 95, 112, 147, 161, 183, 186, 194, 212, 232, 244

Endocrine System, 9, 55, 56, 74

Epilepsy, 38, 90, 99

F

FDA, 125, 221, 225, 228, 229

Fibromyalgia, 91, **140-141**, 258

Fungi, 108, 110, 141, 146, 185, 203, 207

G

Gastritis, 38, 119, **185-186**, 257

Gertsch, J., 21, 22, 24

Glaucoma, 91, **131-134**, 258

Greens, 90, 92, 113, 132, 137, 138, 146, 154, 164, 172, 176, 178, 185, 190, 191, 218, 234

H

Haider, Dr. Paul, 23

Hallucinations, 51, 115, 222

Hallucinogens, 52, 73, 85, 172, 223, 254

Hashish, 34-42, 222, 253
 see also Club des Hashischins

Heart attack, 59, 61, 72, 83-85, 128, 129

Heart disease, 72, 84, 95, **116-127**, 131, 201, 239, 241

Hemp, CO_2 extract of, 13, 105, 106, 122, 182, 208
 fiber, 34, **235-236**
 industrial, 8, 11, 12, 51, 73, 97, 98, 223, 225-229, 236, 237, 251, 254
 medicinal, 87, 154, 170, 176

oil, 91, 102, 112, 117, 124, 129, 130, 150, 176, 225, 237, 238, 240
protein, 241-242
seeds, 7, 32, 33, 52, 53, 131, 155, 156, 235, 241-243
Hepatitis, 177, 257
Heroin, 35, 52, 53, 68, 77, 81, 82, 193, 201, 222, 254
Homeostasis, 11, 26, 28, 56, 165
Hops, 9, 13, 19, 22, 23, 88, 92-95, 118-125, 154, 155, 187, 233
Hormones, 55, 58, 61, 181, 205, 208, 210
Huntington's disease, 69, 166

I

Impotence, 62, 208, 210
Infections, 107, 113, 141, 152, 180, 211, 249
Infectious Agents and Epilepsy, 107
Inflammatory bowel disease, 176
Insomnia, 47, 49, 90, 118-125, 244, 256

J-L

Journal of Clinical Psychiatry, 163
K2, 85
Limonene, 19, 25, 98, 233
Linalool, 25, 233, 241
Liver disease, 177-178
Lyme disease, 186-187, 257, 258

M

Magnesium, 32, 126, 129, 131, 138,

139, 148, 155, 159, 162, 212, 222, 235, 242, 243
Marijuana edibles, 170-172, 217-218, 223
Mellick, Dr. Larry, 43, 44
Memory loss, 91, 115, 195, 256
Migraine headaches, 49, 61, 136-138, 258
Mold, 80, 81, 108, 110, 115-117, 126, 140, 141, 184, 185
Mother Jones, 80, 252
Multiple sclerosis, 53, 91, 105, 113, 161-162, 256
Mycotoxin poisoning, 117
Myrcene, 19, 25, 122, 123

N

Nausea, 43, 48, 50, 101, 102, 126, 180-181, 257
Nervous agitation, 65, 150, 159-161, 208, 256
Nicotine, 82, 202, 249
Nutritional deficiency, 148, 155, 156, 210

O-Q

Obsessive compulsive syndrome, 149-150
Opium, 34, 52, 53, 253
O'Shaughnessy, William B., 37
Oxygen deprivation, 60, 78, 79, 126, 128
Parasites, 107, 110, 112-114, 146, 161, 207
Parkinson's disease, 91, 105, 113, 146-147, 256
Phytochemicals, 8, 26, 38, 145

Plantar fasciitis, **141-142**, 258
Prophet Muhammad, 35

R

Rabies, 38
Radiation, 153, 190-192, 207, 298
Rimonabant, 243
Rosemary, 9, 13, 19, 22, 23, 88, 92-95,
    106, 114, 135-137, 141, 146, 148-
    150, 152, 154-156, 158, 160, 162,
    166, 167, 172, 173, 175, 180, 187,
    190, 191, 203, 204, 206-213, 233,
    247

S

Schizophrenia, 69, 90, 112, **148-149**,
    256
Sedatives, 25, 99, 119, 122, 123
Seizures, 90, 107-110, 112, 114, 116,
    118, 199, 215, 216
Seizure Syndromes, **106-118**
Sesquiterpenes, 10
Sleep apnea, **125-127**, 256
Smokers, 20, 44, 47, 52, 58, 62-64, 67,
    74-76, 84, 132, 170, 202
Spinal disorders, **167-168**, 258
Stillbirths, **59-61**
Stress, 21, 56, 57, 63, 77, 84, 92, 95,
    122, 128, 129, 155, 156, 160, 170,
    181, 186, 198, 206-208, 231, 246,
    256, 258
Stroke, 62, 72, 150, 151, 165, 256
Stroke recovery, **150-152**, 165, 256
Suicide, 63, 73, **168-173**, 224, 244
Sulak, D., 27, 28
SV40, 109, 112

T

Tapeworms, 107
    beef, *Taneia saginata*, 107, 111
    pork, *Taneia solium*, 107, 111
Terpenes, 9, 10, 18-20, 38, 88, 98,
    232-234
Terpenophenolic compounds, 18
Tetrahydrocannabinol, 12, 51, 72
THC,
    toxicity of, 57
    sexual toxicity of, 208-210
    heart damage from, 85, 130
    digestive toxicity of, 102
    nerve cell damage and, 113, 121
    intraoculer pressure and, 132
    tourettes syndrome and, 163
    in Huntington's disease, 166
    in marijuana edibles, 170-172,
        217-218, 223

Tourette's Syndrome, 163, 164

U-V

Ulcers, 185
Vaccines, 107, 108, 145, 146, 152, 201
Varner, Dr. Michael, 59, 60
Vomiting, 43, 49, 102, 180, 181, 215,
    216, 257

W-Z

Yeast infections, See Candida